REEYA GARG
AMRITA AGGARWAL
NEERAJ YADAV

Medical Management Of Tobacco Associated OPMD

REEYA GARG
AMRITA AGGARWAL
NEERAJ YADAV

Medical Management Of Tobacco Associated OPMD

An Interdisciplinary Review of Clinical Approaches and Therapeutic Strategies in Tobacco-Associated OPMDs

LAP LAMBERT Academic Publishing

Cover image: www.ingimage.com

Publisher:
LAP LAMBERT Academic Publishing
is a trademark of
Dodo Books Indian Ocean Ltd. and OmniScriptum S.R.L publishing group

120 High Road, East Finchley, London, N2 9ED, United Kingdom
Str. Armeneasca 28/1, office 1, Chisinau MD-2012, Republic of Moldova, Europe
Managing Directors: Ieva Konstantinova, Victoria Ursu
info@omniscriptum.com

Printed at: see last page
ISBN: 978-620-8-44352-8

ACKNOWLEDGEMENT

This Research work was possible only because of great efforts put by large number of people. It would leave a void in this dissertation, if their efforts are not acknowledged.

First of all, I would like to thank the Almighty god for giving me a good life. I am eternally obliged to lot of kind individuals who have helped me whole heartedly during every step of this research work and have reaffirmed my faith in human nature. I am very grateful to my grandparents Late Sh. GL Garg and Smt. Vimla Devi for their unconditional love and blessings, my parents Mr. Sheetal Garg & Mrs. Bharti Garg , for their patience and support and making me what I am today. Without their support, I would not be able to purse my post-graduation. I would like to convey my heartful gratitude to my Brother Mr. Divyang Garg , Mr. Udit Garg and sister in law Mrs. Ekta Dugar who have been the backbone in every aspect of my life. I would also like to express my gratitude to my uncle and aunt Mr. Vimal Garg and Mrs. Seema Garg.

I am highly obliged for the extensive guidance and assistance rendered to me by my guide Dr. Anshuman Jamdade, Professor and Head of Department of Oral Medicine & Radiology, Mahatma Gandhi Dental College and Hospital, Jaipur. His patience and support helped me to complete this research work under his guidance in the most beautiful manner it could have been. I am fortunate to be under his unlimited source of knowledge, skill and the perfection he desires in his work and sees in his students.

I express my deepest gratitude to Dr. Satyapal Yadav (Professor & Co Guide), Dr.Neeraj Yadav (Professor), Dr. Amrita Aggarwal (Reader) for their expert opinion, motivation and support during the preparation of this study and throughout my post graduate course.
I would like to post my sincere thanks to my seniors Dr Monika Gupta Dr Kanishka Singh, Dr Saurabh Kanawa for being a greatest support & helping hand throughout. I immensely thanks to my seniors Dr Anuja Sharma and Dr Kanupriya Sharma for their constant care, support and stood by me whenever I needed them the most.

I would like to post my sincere thanks to Dr Harsha Patni , Dr Rishika Singh , for their constant care, support and motivation.
In the end I wish to thank all those who have directly and indirectly contributed to the completion of this dissertation.

Dr. Reeya Garg

INDEX

INTRODUCTION

The term "Oral Potentially Malignant Disorders" (OPMDs) was first introduced at the WHO Workshop in 2005, replacing earlier terms like "precancer" and "precancerous lesions." Previously, the WHO in 1978 classified these conditions into "precancerous lesions" "precancerous conditions" The 2005 workshop highlighted that only a minority of OPMDs progress to oral cancer and that cancer could develop in different oral sites, not just where an OPMD is present. Consequently, "potentially malignant" replaced "precancerous," and "lesions" and "conditions" were merged into "disorders" to reflect a broader risk influenced by environmental carcinogens. In 2020, the WHO further refined the definition, emphasizing that OPMDs indicate a statistically increased risk of oral cancer, not only due to the disorder itself but also due to the patient's genetic and molecular predisposition, which increases lifetime susceptibility to malignancy. [2] Oral Potentially Malignant Disorder is a group of disorders of varying etiologies, usually tobacco; characterized by mutagen-associated, spontaneous or hereditary alterations or mutations in the genetic material of oral epithelial cells with or without clinical and micromorphological alterations that may lead to oral squamous cell carcinoma transformation [2] Oral Leukoplakia (OLP) { 0% to 36.4%} , erythroplakia (EP) {14% to over 50%}, Proliferative Verrucous Leukoplakia {43.87% to 65.8%} Oral submucous fibrosis (OSMF) {7 to 13%}, Oral lichen planus (OLP) {0.44% to 3.8% }, actinic keratosis {3.07% to 17%} (AK), discoid lupus erythematosus (DLE) {10-25%}, and palatal lesions among reverse smokers constitute OPMD .[3] It is generally believed that the prevalence of OPMD worldwide varies between 1 and 5 % [4] The potential for malignant transformation among these conditions vary from less than 1 % to as high as 36 % [5] Oral cancer is by far the most common cancer in India; laryngeal cancers are common in the Western world and nasopharyngeal cancers in the Chinese and southeast population [6] Oral squamous cell carcinoma (OSCC) is the most prevalent type of oral cancer, accounting for 90% of all oral, head, and neck cancers· [7]Apart from being possible pre-cursors to oral cancer, OPMD by themselves are usually debilitating conditions having an influence on the quality of life, both in terms of pain and social disability [8]

Tobacco use, genetic pedis-position, Human papilloma-virus (HPV) infection, poor oral hygiene, denture wearing, mouthwash use , dietary factors, low socio economic status, co-morbidities, and genetic disorders UV Light are other associated risk factors for OSCC and OPMD [9]

The malignant transformation process is known to originate from normal mucosa exposed to various risk factors, leading to progressive changes in different subtypes of oral potentially malignant disorders (OPMDs) and ultimately resulting in the development of OSCC. Chronic exposure to alcohol and tobacco disrupts the genetic stability of oral mucosal keratinocytes, affecting genes such as NOTCH1, TP53, EGFR, CDKN2A, and STAT3, which are commonly identified in premalignant lesions and carcinomas. The synergistic mutagenic effects of alcohol and tobacco, along with increased oral mucosal permeability, contribute to alterations in the tumor and immune microenvironment, promoting loss of cell adhesion and facilitating invasion [10]

Tobacco is closely associated with the development of oral potentially malignant lesions (OPML) such as leukoplakia, erythroplakia oral sub-mucous fibrosis, Palatal lesions in reverse smoker's [11] According to the World Health Organization (WHO), 80% of the world's 1.3 billion tobacco users live in low and middle-income countries (LMICs) [6] The majority (90%) of tobacco consumers reside in Southeast Asia [12] Epidemiological studies in India have shown that up to 80% of oral cancer patients are tobacco users. [13] The most widely used products include chewable tobacco leaves, smoking form of tobacco {beedi , hookah, cigarette} Betel quid or PAAN with tobacco, Gutkha, Naswar, Chaini, Misri, [14] The difference of incidence and site-wise distribution of head-and-neck cancer between India and most parts of the world is believed to be due to the difference in tobacco consumption pattern. [15] The likelihood of developing OPMDs was significantly greater in individuals who consumed tobacco in different forms.[16] Malignant Transformation rate in Tobacco associated OPMD include Leukoplakia , Erythroplakia , OSMF , Smoker's Palate is more in comparison to non tobacco associated OPMD [17] Tobacco products contain more than thirty carcinogens [18]. The ingredients include sun-cured unprocessed or processed tobacco of Nicotiana tabacum and Nicotiana rustica species. Tobacco-specific N-nitrosamines (TSNAs) – N-nitrosonornicotine, 4-(methylnitrosamino)-1-(3-pyridyl)-1-butanone, and N-nitrosamino acids – are the most prevalent strong carcinogens in smokeless tobacco , along with heavy metals such as nickel, cadmium, chromium, and copper [19] The carcinogens cause the formation of DNA adducts and subsequent mutations in K-ras, p53 and other genes, leading to uncontrolled cell growth. Other changes, including chronic local inflammation, oxidative stress and formation of reactive oxygen species, may also contribute to tumor promotion [20] A strong correlation was identified between tobacco use and the prevalence of OPMDs.[21] Notably, 11.4% of tobacco users were diagnosed with OPMDs, compared to just 1.4% of non-tobacco users. [21]

Management is usually based on disease severity and focuses on reversing or alleviating these signs and symptoms, stopping the disease progressing, and minimizing the risk of malignant transformation [22] . Medical management provide a non-invasive, cost-effective approach that preserves oral structure and function. It effectively manages multifocal lesions, lowers recurrence risk by addressing underlying causes, and is ideal for high-risk patients, providing both preventive and supportive benefits. The current protocol for managing the condition can be divided into two broad groups: conservative treatment and surgical therapy Conservative treatment includes Tobacco cessation therapies chemo preventive agents, topical tretinoin/isotretinoin, topical bleomycin, 13-cis-retinoic acid and photodynamic therapy.[23] Steroids , Interferon c , Immunized milk ,Placental extracts , Levamisole , Colchicine , Pentoxyphylline , Buflomedil hydrochloride , Nylidrin ß-carotene , Lycopene , Tea pigments , Vitamins and mineral supplements ,Hyaluronidase , Chymotrypsin , Collagenase Anti-TGF b drugs, , copper chelators , Borneol , Garlic extracts , Oxitard , Danuxan Koukung , Aloe vera ,Turmeric or curcumin longa Linn [24] Conservative treatment is often preferred over surgical treatment due to its less invasive nature, lower risk of complications, and cost-effectiveness. Additionally, it usually results in quicker recovery times and aligns with patient preferences.

TOBACCO AND ITS ROLE IN OPMD

Tobacco refers to the plant species Nicotiana tabacum, which is cultivated for its leaves, which are dried and processed for various uses, particularly smoking, chewing, or snuffing. The primary active ingredient in tobacco is nicotine, a highly addictive substance. Nicotin causes Relaxation during stress, Improved attention, learning, reaction time and problem solving; Reduced hunger etc. Tobacco products come in various forms, including cigarettes, cigars, pipe tobacco, chewing tobacco, and snuff. Tobacco is used in various ways, which include smoking forms as (Beedis, Cigarettes, Cigar, Cheerot, Chhutta, Dhumti, Hookli, Hookah, Chillum, Pipe), smokeless forms (Pan, Pan masala, Mawa, Khaini, Mainpuri tobacco, Chewing tobacco, Snuff), tobacco products for application (Mishri, Gul, Lal dantmanjan, Bajjar, Gudakhu, Creamy snuff, Areca nut preparation (Areca nut, Supari, Meetha mawa). In India, Beedi is most popular form of tobacco smoking followed by cigarette smoking. Pan with tobacco is major form of chewing tobacco.[28] .India is the second largest consumer of tobacco in the world. The prevalence of tobacco use among men has been reported to be high in most parts of the country (generally exceeding 50%). Its use is more common in rural areas as compared to urban areas.[25]

Tobacco use causes a wide range of major diseases which impact nearly every organ of the body. Tobacco-related illnesses such as cancer and cardiovascular and respiratory diseases are already major problems. Tobacco use is a risk factor for six of the eight leading causes of death in the world.

TYPES OF TOBACCO [26]

SMOKELESS TOBACCO

Smokeless tobacco is usually consumed orally or nasally, without burning or combustion. There are two main types of smokeless tobacco: snuff and chewing tobacco.

1. **DRY SNUFF**- Dry snuff is powdered tobacco that is inhaled through the nose and absorbed through the nasal mucosa or taken orally. Once widespread, particularly in Europe, the use of dry snuff is in decline.
   - Most Prevalent: Europe

1. **MOIST SNUFF** - Moist snuff is a small amount of ground tobacco held in the mouth between the cheek and gum. Manufacturers are increasingly pre packaging moist snuff into small paper or cloth packets to make the product more convenient. Other moist snuff products are known as khaini, snus, shammaah, nass, or naswa.
   - Most Prevalent: Worldwide

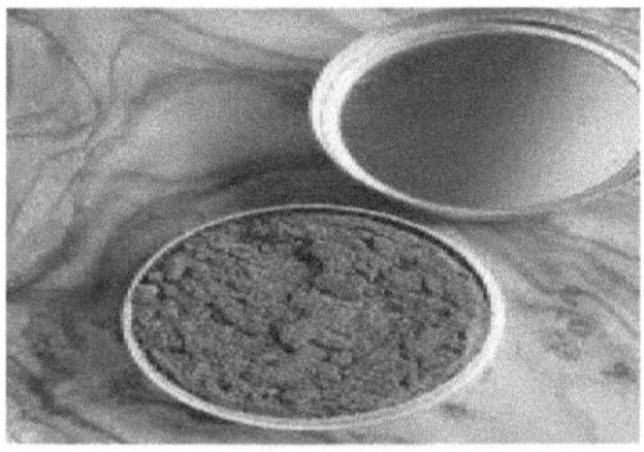

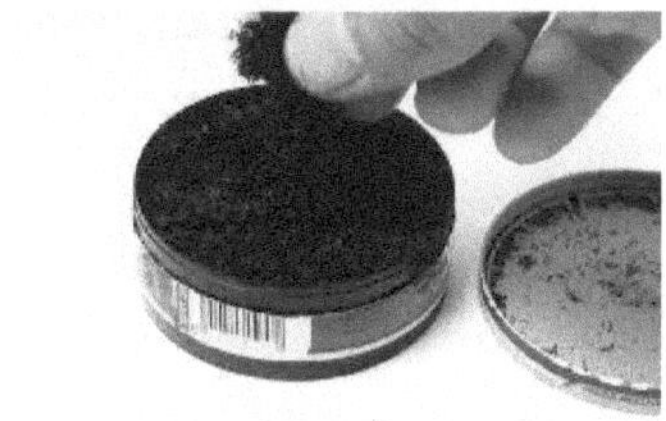

2. **CHEWING TOBACCO** - Oral smokeless tobacco products are placed in the mouth, cheek, or inner lip and sucked (dipped) or chewed. Tobacco pastes or powders are similarly used, placed on the gums or teeth. Sometimes referred to as "spit tobacco" because users spit out the built-up tobacco juices and saliva, this mode of tobacco consumption became associated with American baseball players during the twentieth century. The tobacco industry exploited these sports heroes to market their tobacco products to youth. Smokeless tobacco causes cancer in humans and leads to nicotine addiction similar to that produced by cigarette smoking. There are many varieties of smokeless tobacco, including plug, loose- leaf, chimo, toombak, gutkha, and twist. Pan masala or betel quid consists of tobacco, areca nuts (Areca catechu), slaked lime (calcium hydroxide), sweeteners, and flavoring agents wrapped in a betel leaf (Piper betel). There are endless varieties of pan masala, including kaddipudi, hogesoppu, gundi, kadapam, zarda, pattiwala, kiwam, and mishri.

- Most Prevalent: India

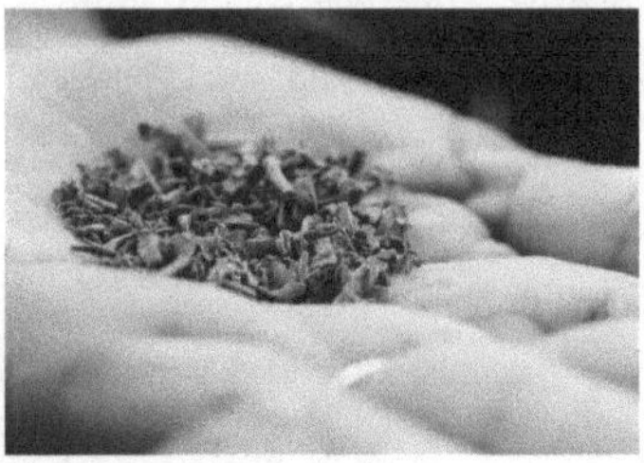

SMOKING TOBACCO

Tobacco smoking is the act of burning dried or cured leaves of the tobacco plant and inhaling the smoke. Combustion releases biochemically active compounds in tobacco, such as nicotine and TSNA, and allows them to be absorbed through the lungs.

1. **ROLL-YOUR-OWN (RYO)**-cigarettes are cigarettes hand-filled by the smoker from fine-cut, loose tobacco rolled in a cigarette paper. RYO cigarette smokers are exposed to high concentrations of tobacco particulates, tar, nicotine, and tobacco-specific nitrosamines (TSNAs), and are at increased risk for developing cancers of the mouth, pharynx, larynx, lung, and esophagus.

- Most Prevalent: Europeand New Zealand

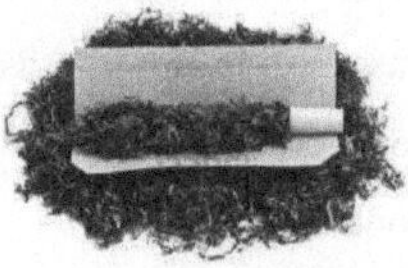

1. **MANUFACTURED CIGARETTES** - are the most commonly consumed tobacco products worldwide. They consist of shredded or reconstituted tobacco, processed with hundreds of chemicals and rolled into a paper-wrapped cylinder. Usually tipped with a cellulose acetate filter, they are lit at one end and inhaled through the other.

- Most Prevalent: Worldwide

1. **CIGARS-** Cigars are made of air-cured and fermented tobaccos with a tobacco-leaf wrapper. The long aging and fermentation process produces

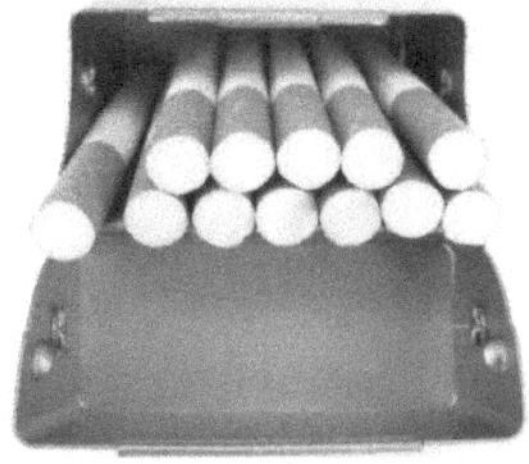

high concentrations of carcinogenic compounds that are released on combustion. The concentrations of toxins and irritants in cigars are higher than in cigarettes. Cigars come in many shapes and sizes, from cigarette-sized cigarillos to double coronas, cheroots, stumpen, chuttas, and dhumtis. In reverse chutta and dhumti smoking, the ignited end of the cigar is placed inside the mouth.

- Most Prevalent: Worldwide

1. **BIDIS-** consist of a small amount of sun-dried, flaked tobacco handwrapped

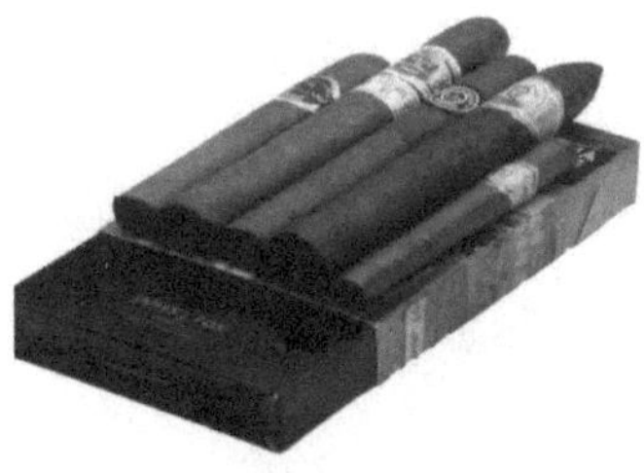

in dried temburni or tendu leaf (Diospyros sp.) and tied with string. Despite their small size, bidis deliver more tar and carbon monoxide than manufactured cigarettes because users are forced to puff harder to keep bidis lit. Bidis are found throughout South Asia and are the most heavily consumed smoked tobacco products in India.

- Most Prevalent: South Asia

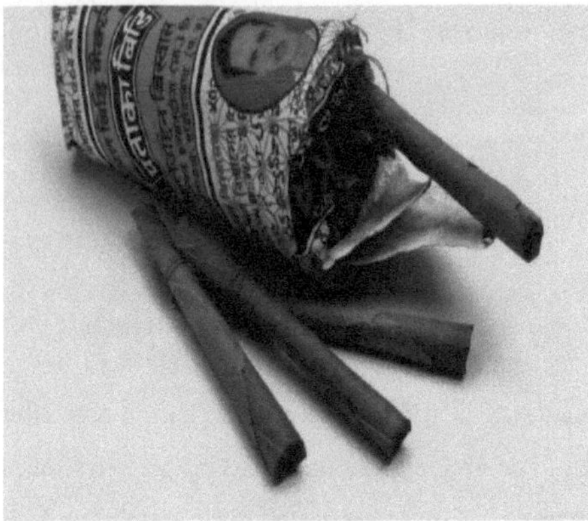

2. **KRETEKS** - Kreteks are clove-flavored cigarettes widely smoked in Indonesia. They may contain a wide range of exotic flavorings and eugenol, which has an anesthetic effect, allowing for deeper and more harmful smoke inhalation.
   - Most Prevalent: Indonesia

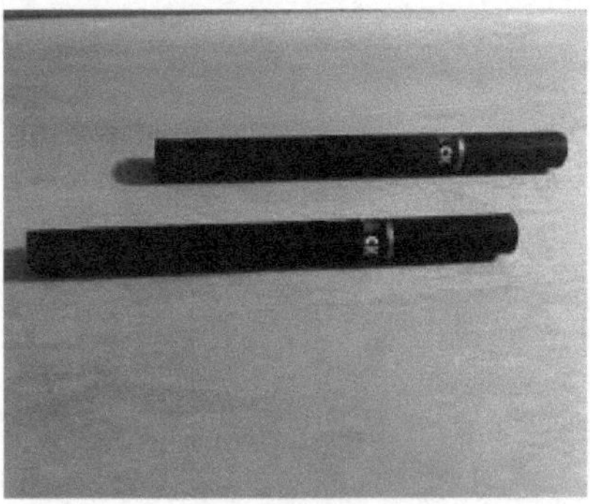

3. **WATER PIPES** -Water pipes, also known as shisha, hookah, narghile, or hubble-bubble, operate by water filtration and indirect heat. Flavored tobacco is burned in a smoking bowl covered with foil and coal. The smoke is cooled by filtration through a basin of water and consumed through a hose and mouthpiece.
    - Most Prevalent: North Africa, the Mediterranean region, and parts of Asia

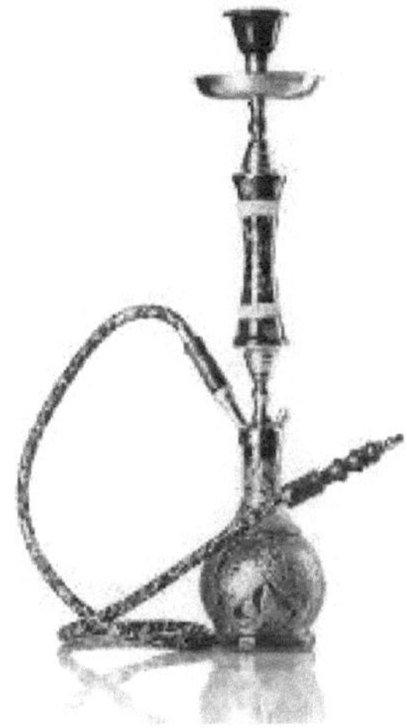

4. **PIPES** - Pipes are made of briar, slate, clay, or other substances. Tobacco is placed in the bowl, and the smoke is inhaled through the stem. In Southeast Asia, clay pipes known as sulpa, chillum, and hookli are widely used.
    - Most Prevalent: Worldwide

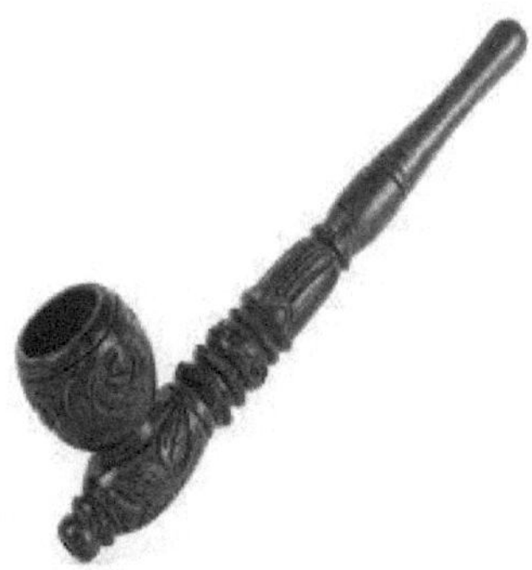

5. **STICKS** - Sticks are made from sun-cured tobacco and wrapped in cigarette paper—for example, hand-rolled brus.
   - Most Prevalent: Papua New Guinea

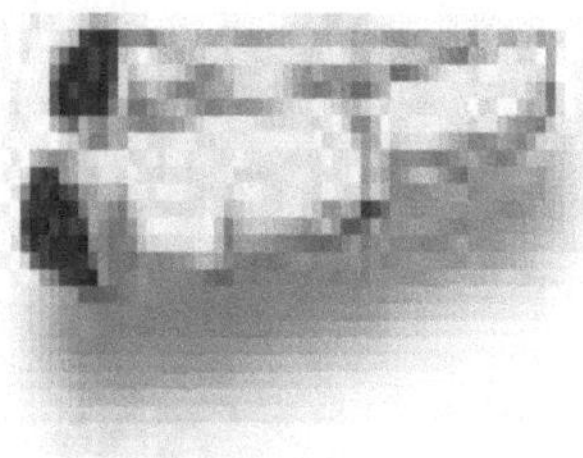

Smokeless tobacco (SLT) use is considered as a major risk factor for OPMD. It is important to mention that around 80% of cases of oral malignancies can be directly attributed to tobacco consumption. [27] . OPMDs such as leukoplakia, oral submucous fibrosis (OSMF), tobacco pouch keratosis, and smoker's palate were observed in 11.4% of individuals who used tobacco.[28]

CARCINOGENIC COMPOUNDS IN TOBACCO

Smokeless tobacco contains chemical carcinogens such as benzo[a]pyrene, nicotine, and tobacco specific N-nitrosamines, which can induce dysplastic changes in the oral mucosa. Chronic intraoral placement of smokeless tobacco leads to chronic irritation, triggering the deposition of excess fibrin-like material and an increase in keratin production, characteristic of lesions like smokeless tobacco keratosis. Leukoplakia and erythroplakia, both clinically diagnostic terms for oral lesions, can also arise from the carcinogenic effects of tobacco and serve as visible indicators of tissue damage and potential malignant transformation [29] In the case of OSMF, while areca nut-chewing is identified as the primary causative agent, the chewing of smokeless tobacco significantly contributes to its development. The chronic exposure to carcinogens and irritants presents in smokeless tobacco exacerbates fibrotic changes in the oral submucosa, leading to the characteristic stiffness and limited mouth opening associated with OSMF [30]

Smokeless tobacco (SLT) use is a major risk factor for OPMDs. Around 80% of oral malignancies can be directly attributed to tobacco consumption. OPMDs such as leukoplakia, oral submucous fibrosis (OSMF), tobacco pouch keratosis, and smoker's palate are observed in 11.4% of individuals who use tobacco.

Smokeless tobacco contains chemical carcinogens such as:

- **Benzo[a]pyrene**
- **Nicotine**
- **Tobacco-specific N-nitrosamines (TSNAs)**

These compounds induce dysplastic changes in the oral mucosa. Chronic intraoral placement of smokeless tobacco leads to chronic irritation, triggering excess fibrin-like material deposition and increased keratin production, characteristic of lesions like smokeless tobacco keratosis.

Leukoplakia and erythroplakia are clinically diagnostic terms for oral lesions arising from tobacco's carcinogenic effects. These serve as visible indicators of tissue damage and potential malignant transformation.

In the case of OSMF, while areca nut chewing is the primary cause, smokeless tobacco significantly contributes to its development. Chronic exposure to carcinogens and irritants in smokeless tobacco exacerbates fibrotic changes in the oral submucosa, leading to stiffness and limited mouth opening, characteristic of OSMF.

CLASSIFICATION OF ORAL POTENTIALLY MALIGNANT DISORDER

Oral potentially malignant disorders (OPMDs) are defined as a group of disorders where the clinical presentation may precede the diagnosis of an oral squamous cell carcinoma (OSCC) .

The term OPMDs was first introduced at the World Health Organisation (WHO) Workshop in 2005, leading to the disuse of many other terms previously used including 'precancer', 'epithelial precursor lesions', 'premalignant', 'precancerous', and 'intra-epithelial lesion [1]

'Precancer' is one of the oldest terms initially described in 1805 to describe benign diseases that may develop into invasive malignancy if followed over a long period of time . In 1978, the term 'precancerous lesions' was adopted by the WHO working group, with a division into precancerous lesions (e.g. leukoplakia, erythroplakia) and precancerous conditions (e.g. oral submucous fibrosis, actinic keratosis, oral lichen planus, or discoid lupus erythematosus) [31]

In the WHO 2005 OPMD Workshop, the working group made two observations. The first was that this association or risk is potential during the lifetime of the patient, and only a minority progress to oral cancer (and not all as a 'precancerous' terminology would suggest). The second was that an oral cancer could not only appear in the same location of a previous OPMD, but also in another location of the oral cavity of a patient with a lesion or condition identified as an OPMD [1]

with significant changes in terminology related to oral cancer risk were introduced [32]:

1. The term "potentially malignant" replaced "precancerous" to better describe mucosal abnormalities that indicate a risk of developing oral cancer, but not necessarily.
2. The terms "lesions" and "conditions" were merged into "disorders," acknowledging that oral cancers could develop from these mucosal alterations anywhere in the oral cavity. This reflects the impact of environmental carcinogens on the upper aero-digestive tract, with disorders indicating a potential increased risk of oral cancer elsewhere in the oral cavity.

The WHO Collaborating Centre Consensus Workshop on OPMDs in 2020, updated the definition of an OPMD as 'any oral mucosal abnormality that is associated with a statistically increased risk of developing oral cancer' It has put an emphasis not only directly to the disorder itself, but also to the patient who may carry genomic and other molecular abnormalities in the oral mucosa, promoting the existence of an OPMD and, potentially, an oral cancer Therefore, patients diagnosed with OPMDs have an increased susceptibility to develop oral cancer in their lifetime [1]

Classification [1]

1. Leukoplakia
2. Proliferative verrucous leukoplakia
3. Erythroplakia
4. Oral Submucous Fibrosis (OSMF)
5. Oral lichen planus
6. Actinic Keratosis/Actinic Cheilitis
7. Palatal lesions in reverse smokers
8. Oral lupus erythematosus
9. Dyskeratosis congenita
CONDITIONS NEWLY ADDED IN 2020 CLASSIFICATION

1. Oral lichenoid Lesions (OLL)
2. Oral graft versus host disease (OGVHD)

Leukoplakia

WHO Collaborating Centre for Oral Cancer in 2020 defined Leukoplakia as 'A predominantly white plaque of questionable risk having excluded (other) known diseases or disorders that carry no increased risk for cancer. [33]

Classification of Leukoplakia

Homogenous leukoplakia	Non-homogenous leukoplakia
• Uniform flat and thin white plaque/patch with well-defined margins, smooth surface associated with shallow cracks/fissures. Cannot be scraped off.	Speckled: mixed white and red color • Nodular: small polypoid outgrowths, rounded, red or white nodules • Verrucous or exophytic: wrinkled or corrugated surface. • Cannot be scraped off.

Proliferative Verrucous Leukoplakia

Proliferative verrucous leukoplakia (PVL) was first defined in 1985, when Hansen and colleagues first described a particular form of leukoplakia, characterised by slow-growth and persistence, with a tendency to spread, become multifocal, and exophytic or wart-like with time [34]More recently, alternative terms 'Proliferative Multifocal Leukoplakia' and 'Proliferative Leukoplakia' have been suggested. 'Proliferative Multifocal Leukoplakia' was proposed by Aguirre-Urizar, to emphasize the proliferative and multifocal nature rather than the verrucous appearance [35]'Proliferative Leukoplakia', proposed by Villa and colleagues, was based on data demonstrating an absence of a verrucous appearance in almost 40% of cases.

In 2020, the Working Group of the WHO Collaborating Centre for Oral Cancer acknowledged that 'despite the imperfection of the term PVL to capture an expanded group of patients with multifocal disease, the term is widely reported, and the Working Group recommended retaining this term'. The same group proposed the following definition: 'a progressive, persistent, and irreversible disorder characterised by the presence of multiple leukoplakias that frequently become warty'

PVL can be considered a distinct form of oral leukoplakia (OL) characterised by multifocal lesions, progressive clinical course and changes in clinical appearance and histopathologic features . However, such a position to classify PVL as a separate entity is not universally agreed, since large, widespread leukoplakias, and not only PVLs, carry a distinct risk of malignant transformation .

Erythroplakia

The World Health Organisation (WHO) originally defined erythroplakia as 'any lesion of the oral mucosa that presents as bright red velvety plaques which cannot be characterized clinically or pathologically as any other recognizable condition. [36]

Oral Submucous Fibrosis

A chronic, insidious disease that affects the oral mucosa, initially resulting in loss of fibro elasticity of the lamina propria and as the disease advances, results in fibrosis of the lamina propria and the submucosa of the oral cavity along with epithelial atrophy. [37]

Classification of oral submucous fibrosis based on clinical parameters[38]

Stage 1: Mild Any features of the disease (BS, depapillation, blanching or leathery OM) and MO >35mm.
Stage 2: Moderate Above features + MO 20–35mm.
Stage 3: Severe Above features + MO < 20mm.
Stage 4A: OSMF + other potentially malignant disorder evident clinically.
Stage 4B: OSMF with any grade of OED on biopsy. Stage 5: OSMF with features of OSCC.

Palatal lesions in Reverse Smoker's

In 2020, the World Health Organization (WHO) collaborating Centre for oral cancer, defined palatal lesions in reverse smokers (PLRS) as 'white and / or red patches affecting the hard palate in reverse smokers, frequently stained with nicotine [37]

Grading system for these lesions:

• Grade 0 in which no palatal changes are observed
• Grade 1 in which mild palatal changes are observed such as 'red circular areas over a slightly raised blanched mucosa of the glandular zone of the hard palate.'
• Grade 2 represent moderate palatal changes such as 'papules of 2-4mm with central umbilication less than 2mm of diameter. Moderate changes include hyper keratinization and premalignant changes like leukoplakia.'
• Grade 3 represent severe palatal changes such as 'papules greater than 4-5mm in size with central umbilicus 2-4 mm in size or characterized by crater like ulcerations surrounded by keratinization'. • Grade 4 lesions represent palatal carcinoma

PREVALENCE AND DEMOGRAPHIC TRENDS

The worldwide prevalence of OPMD had been estimated at 4.47% (95% CI = 2.43–7.08). This may vary between populations and is higher in Asian populations and males.[1]

The majority of patients with OPMDs are middle-aged or elderly. [39]

Ethnicity and cultural habits influence the type and pattern of OPMDs reported in specific populations due to the dominance of particular risk factors. For example, betel quid/areca nut chewing habits are widely prevalent in South Asian populations resulting in a greater prevalence of OPMDs. [1]

Oral leukoplakia is commonly diagnosed in middle aged to elderly patients. It is globally more commonly identified in males. OL is six times more common among smokers than non-smokers OL rarely occurs in the first two decades of life, and the condition is usually diagnosed after the fourth decade. OL may arise anywhere in the oral cavity and may be uni- or multifocal However, in Western industrialised populations, the most common sites of involvement are the lateral border of the tongue and floor of the mouth In Asian populations, due to the frequent consumption of betel quid, the buccal mucosa and the labial mucosa are often affected The prevalence of OL varies significantly with geographical variations due to different risk factors, such as betel nut chewing in South East Asia. However, OL is associated with various risk factors, similar to those observed in oral cancer, such as tobacco (both smoked and smokeless), heavy alcohol consumption, betel quid chewing (especially in South Asian countries) and, for lesions involving the lip, ultraviolet (UV) light exposure. Alcohol consumption is an independent risk factor [5]. It has been established that these factors may have an etiological role in the development of OL in more than 75% of the affected individuals Leukoplakias without a known cause are termed 'idiopathic leukoplakias' Moreover, immunosuppression (e.g. HIV/AIDS, post-organ transplantation), personal or family history of cancer (60%–70%) and selected syndromes (e.g. dyskeratosis congenita, Fanconi anaemia), may be considered risk factors for OL Leukoplakia which develops in a patient with no pre-disposing factors is considered to have un underlying genetic basis for development Several studies have evaluated the role of human papillomavirus (HPV) in the development of OL and a possible correlation has been identified However, the aetiological role of HPV in OL and OSCC development remains controversial .[40]

Oral leukoplakia is more commonly found in men 40 years of age or older with higher prevalence in men and women over 70 [41].

The overall prevalence of OL is estimated to range between 1.5% and 2.6% PVL is less common than standard leukoplakia and data on its prevalence is not available [42]

PVL is associated with the highest incidence of oral cancer amongst OPMDs, either verrucous carcinoma or squamous cell carcinoma Approximately 61% of patients with PVL develop oral cancer over an average period of 7.4 years, though a recent systematic review estimated malignant transformation occurs in 49.5% (CI 26.7%-72.4%) of PVL cases. The annual incidence is estimated to be 10.0% per year [42]

Multiple primary carcinomas of gingival sites have been reported in the literature in patients affected by PVL, evidenced in recent case series. PVL is associated with an overall mortality of 40% [43]

There is a lack of large-scale epidemiological studies investigating the prevalence of oral erythroplakia The prevalence rate varies from approximately 0.02 to 2%. A large-scale study (500) completed on hospital inpatients in India found a prevalence of 0.6% The prevalence amongst a similar sized study in Saudi Arabia (559) was 0.7% An Irish study consisting of 210 addiction treatment center residents found a prevalence as high as 1.9%. Population-based samples have found considerably lower prevalence rates. Studies involving larger samples with more equal gender distribution completed in Brazil and India have found a prevalence of 0.3% and 0.24%, respectively Prevalence of oral erythroplakia is higher in middle-aged and older adults, when reported [44] It is widely accepted that the prevalence of erythroplakia is less than other OPMDs and oral leukoplakia [45] There appears to be no gender predilection, despite earlier studies reporting a male predominance Erythroplakia appears to occur mainly in middle aged and elderly A recent systematic review assessing oral leukoplakia and erythroplakia in younger patients found there was a lack of studies to comment but found the frequency of oral leukoplakia to be lower in younger patients (patients younger than 40 years of age) There is no known geographical distribution of erythroplakia, however, the prevalence is observably higher in populations with a preexisting smoking and betel nut chewing habit.

Oral submucous fibrosis (OSMF) predominantly affects the Indian subcontinent and Southeast Asia, including countries like India, Taiwan, China, and Sri Lanka, but has also been reported globally, including in South Africa, Saudi Arabia, and Asian populations in developed countries. In 1996, an estimated 2.5 million cases were reported worldwide. Symptoms typically manifest in the 4th–5th decades of life, though cases have occurred in children as young as 11. The condition shows a female preponderance for unknown reasons. [46]

Reverse smoking is a smoking habit observed around the world, however, there is a distinct lack of epidemiological studies evaluating the geographic distribution. Reverse smoking is most frequently observed in warm and tropical climates in the developing world, in countries such as Columbia, Venezuela, Panama and India [6]The habit has also been observed in the developed world, for example it is known to be common on the Italian island of Sardinia. In India, reverse smoking appears to be a traditional habit amongst older woman in the southern state of Andhra Pradesh [6]. The type of cigarette used in these areas are often called chutta. A chutta is a coarse preparation of cheroot of varying length which can be prepared by the consumer or in factories. A study investigating the psychosocial factors associated with reverse smoking found that the habit is derived or inherited maternally or from other people in the family or social circle. The study found a profound psychological etiology as there is no apparent physical benefit to perpetuating the habit [47]

A recent systematic review reported an OPMD overall malignant transformation rate of 7.9% (99%CI 4.9% 11.5%) although with high heterogeneity test values

Risk Factors for Progression to malignancy

Prevalence in South Central Asia

Oral cancer has a high predilection in South Central Asia, particularly in India, where it is the second most common cancer among males and the fifth among females.

Morbidity and Mortality

Oral cancer represents a significant health problem globally due to its morbidity and mortality. The 5-year survival rate is about 50%, especially in developing countries, with a higher death rate in males compared to females [48]

Contributing Factors to Mortality

Mortality remains a challenging problem due to:

- Lifestyle habits
- Quality and access to medical assistance
- Health education of the population

- Prevention of OPMDs (Oral Potentially Malignant Disorders)

Avoidable factors such as tobacco and alcohol are involved in 90% of cases, with a synergistic contribution [49].

Pathogenesis and Malignant Transformation

Starting Point of Malignant Transformation:

Malignant transformation begins in the normal mucosa exposed to various risk factors, leading to the progressive modification in different subtypes of OPMDs and, finally, the development of OSCC (Oral Squamous Cell Carcinoma).

Genetic Alterations

Chronic exposure to alcohol and tobacco alters the genetic stability of oral mucosa keratinocytes, involving genes such as:

- NOTCH1
- TP53
- EGFR
- CDKN2A
- STAT3

These genes are commonly found in OPMDs [50].

Mutagenic Effects

Synergistic mutagenic effects and an increase in oral mucosa permeability by alcohol and tobacco lead to the alteration of the tumor and immune microenvironment, promoting cell adhesion loss and invasion [51].

Malignant Transformation Rates of OPMDs

The rate at which patients with OPMDs present with oral malignancy (malignant transformation rate) varies worldwide and is closely related to:

- The type of disorder

- Clinical, pathological, or molecular factors (including type, color, location, size, gender, and the presence and grade of dysplasia) [52].

Specific Malignant Transformation Rates

A recent systematic review reported an overall malignant transformation rate of 7.9% for OPMDs, with specific rates for subgroups:

- Leukoplakia: 9.5%
- Lichen Planus: 1.4%
- Oral Lichenoid Lesions: 3.8%
- Oral Submucous Fibrosis: 5.2%
- Oral Erythroplakia: 33.1%
- Proliferative Verrucous Leukoplakia: 49.5% [1].

Importance of Early Detection and Management

Improved knowledge and better detection of OPMDs are crucial to:

- Provide the best management
- Improve the patient's quality of life
- Ensure close follow-up of these patients, facilitating prevention and early diagnosis of invasive carcinoma involving the oral mucosa.

PATHOGENESIS AND MOLECULAR MECHANISMS

Oral leukoplakia (OL) shares several risk factors with oral cancer, including both smoked and smokeless tobacco, heavy alcohol consumption, betel quid chewing (particularly in South Asia), and UV light exposure for lip lesions. Alcohol is an independent risk factor. These elements contribute to OL's etiology in over 75% of cases. Leukoplakia without an identified cause is known as 'idiopathic leukoplakia'. Additionally, immunosuppression (e.g., HIV/AIDS, post-transplantation), a personal or family cancer history, and certain syndromes (e.g., dyskeratosis congenita, Fanconi anemia) are potential risk factors. Leukoplakia in patients without predisposing factors likely has a genetic basis. Studies indicate a potential link between human papillomavirus (HPV) and OL, though HPV's role in OL and oral squamous cell carcinoma (OSCC) development remains debated.[53]

The etiology of PVL remains unknown. PVL is more common in elderly females without a racial predilection The putative role of human papillomavirus (HPV) has not yet been established . The reported HPV prevalence in PVL ranges from 0-88% based on the results from studies with small patient numbers. A study investigating the prevalence of HPV in 58 patients showed no significant differences between patients affected by PVL and those with conventional OL (24% versus 25%)[54]

Etiopathogenesis of erythroplakia is poorly understood. The factors are primarily betel quid chewing, tobacco chewing, tobacco smoking and alcohol consumption . Other implicated possible etiological factors include BMI and nutritional status . Human papillomavirus (HPV) has also been elucidated as a possible contributory factor or etiological cofactor. However, there is a paucity of research in the area and the associations are based on observational cross-sectional studies [55]

Oral submucous fibrosis (OSMF) is mainly caused by chewing areca nut, also known as betel nut, with development depending on the frequency and duration of chewing. This habit is prevalent in the Indian subcontinent and increasingly common in Western communities due to migration. Areca nut preparations may contain tobacco and other carcinogens. Areca nut itself has cytotoxic and genotoxic properties due to tannins and alkaloids.

Slaked lime in areca nut preparations contains arsenic. Areca nut is considered divine in Hinduism and believed to have medicinal properties, including improved oral hygiene, halitosis reduction, and glycemic control. Arecoline, a byproduct of areca nut metabolism, crosses the blood-brain barrier, contributing to its addictive potential and euphoric effects. It is classified as a Group 1 carcinogen by the International Agency for Research on Cancer.

Genetic predisposition to OSMF may be linked to certain HLA subtypes and haplotypes. Malnutrition, anemia, and hematinic deficiencies can lead to oral mucosa atrophy and increased collagen synthesis. Capsaicin from chili peppers may cause hypersensitivity reactions contributing to fibrosis. OSMF is characterized by abnormal collagen deposition. Areca alkaloids stimulate fibroblast proliferation, while tannins inhibit collagenase activity, leading to resistant type 3 collagen buildup. Arecoline suppresses T-cell activity, and copper enhances lysyl oxidase, increasing collagen and elastin cross-linking. The activation of TGF-Beta is key in increasing collagen production and fibrosis.[56]

Continuous exposure of the palatal mucosa to high temperatures in reverse smoking causes thermal injury. This, combined with combustion products, leads to a higher frequency of palatal lesions compared to conventional smoking. The lips act as a seal, prolonging contact time. The carcinogenic effects of cigarette smoking are well documented. Thermal injury and prolonged contact with carcinogens result in changes to the palatal mucosa.[57]

CLINICAL PRESENTATION AND DIAGNOSIS

Clinically, leukoplakia shows a wide range of variable features in appearance (white, red, and mixed white and red, plaque/plateau granular, atrophic) texture (smooth, corrugated, verrucous granular, soft, firm or hard), and size and shape.

Leukoplakia is generally asymptomatic and are often identified during routine general examination . Homogenous leukoplakia is typically asymptomatic . Symptoms are rare, and if present, are usually associated with the non-homogeneous forms which may show focal superficial ulceration In these cases, the symptoms more frequently reported are discomfort, tingling, and sensitivity to touch, hot beverages, or spicy foods.

The term erythroleukoplakia identifies lesions characterized by mixed white and red color and it should not be confused with the term erythroplakia, which should only be used to describe lesions that are uniformly red.

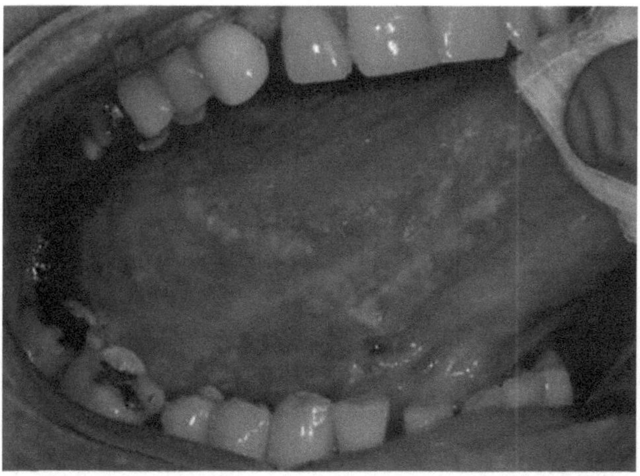

Homogenous Leukoplakia

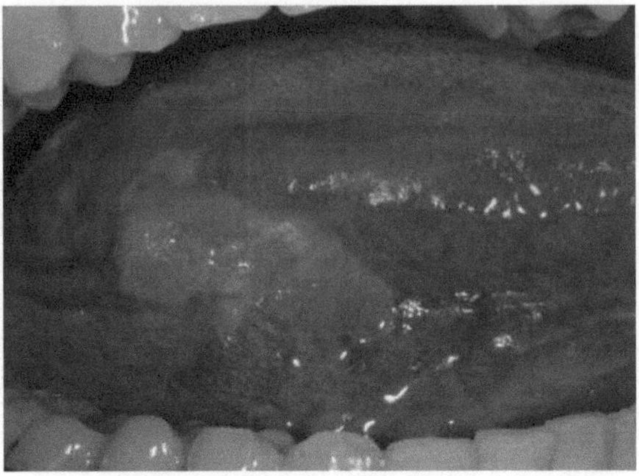

Non-Homogenous Leukoplakia

Oral proliferative verrucous leukoplakia (PVL), a subset of non-homogenous leukoplakia, may be defined as a distinct form of multifocal leukoplakia characterized by a progressive clinical course and changing in clinical appearance and histopathologic features .PVL often presents as one or more leukoplakia, eventually presenting in multiple locations with gradual spread of an individual focus or resulting from fusion over time of several adjacent foci. [58]

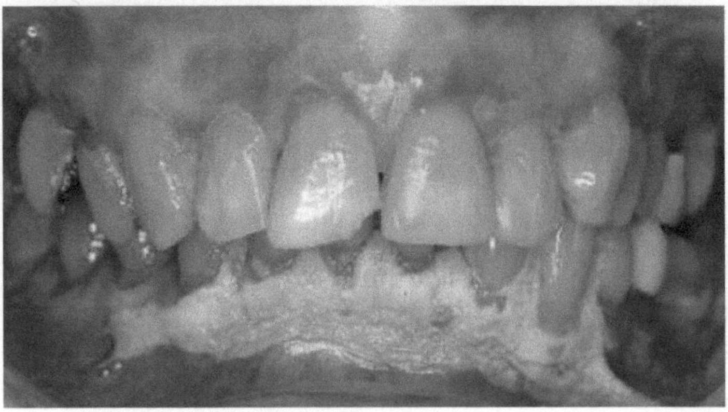

Dense PVL affecting the buccal gingiva in the lower anterior sextant, with nodular components, a speckled patch can also be seen in the lower left buccal sulcus.

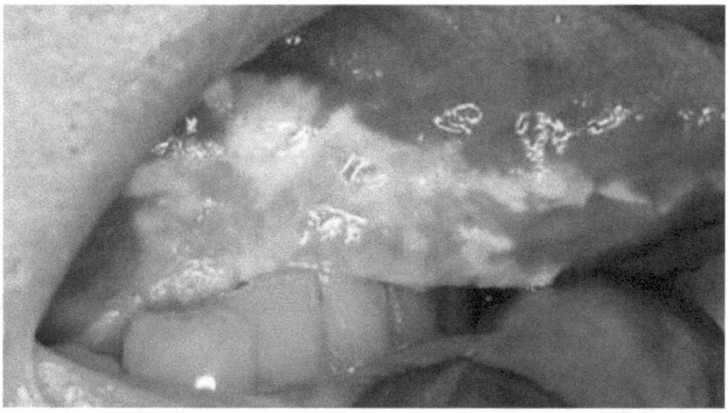

A dense multifocal area of PVL on the encompassing the right lateral tongue.

PVL clinical presentation Multiple, thick, white patches in more than two different oral sites, frequently found on the gingiva, alveolar processes, and palate Majority of the lesion presents a verrucous pattern Lesions spread and coalesce during development Recurrence in a previously treated area

Erythroplakia: [59]

- Appears as fiery red macules or patches with a soft, velvety texture.
- Typically soft to the touch, with induration (hardness) usually only observed in malignant cases.
- Lesions are irregular in outline but well-defined.
- Surface may occasionally appear granular.
- Usually asymptomatic, but patients may report non-specific soreness, burning, or metallic taste.

Erythroleukoplakia:

- Red areas show atrophy or thinning of the epithelium and may have irregular margins.
- More commonly symptomatic than erythroplakia.
- Affects areas like the floor of the mouth, ventral tongue, soft palate, tonsillar fauces, and buccal mucosa.
- Lesions are typically small (less than 1.5 cm) but can be larger (>4 cm).
- Rarely affects multiple sites.

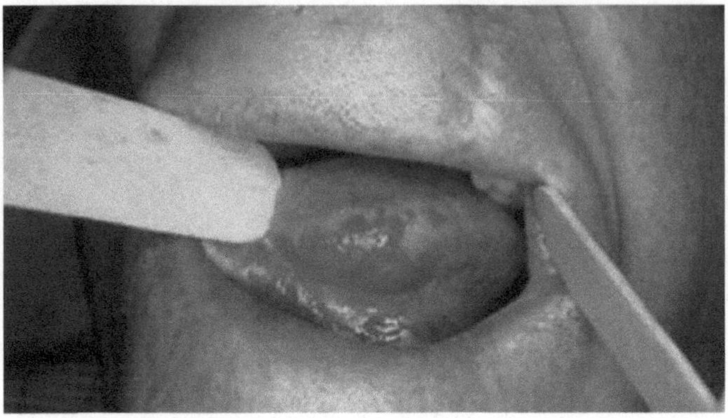

Erythroplakia

Oral Submucous Fibrosis (OSMF) is clinically categorized into four stages by More (2012):[60]

1. **Eruptive Phase:**
    - Vesicle formation
    - Burning sensation and discomfort in the oral cavity
    - Changes in oral mucosa texture, losing suppleness
    - Pallor and blanching of the mucosa
    - Mucosal petechiae, melanotic mucosal pigmentation, mucosal ulceration, erythematous areas
2. **Fibrotic Phase:**
    - Fibrosis in vesicles and ulcers upon healing
    - Vertical and circular palpable fibrous bands in buccal mucosa and/or oropharynx, with or without stomatitis
    - Thinner bands in early stages
3. **Advanced Fibrosis:**
    - Palpable fibrous bands in any part of the oral cavity, with or without stomatitis
4. **Malignant Transformation:**
    - Development of potentially malignant disorders or frank oral squamous cell carcinoma
    - Trismus, gingival depigmentation, atrophic uvula, depapillation of the tongue
    - Facial aesthetic changes like sinking cheeks

- Severe cases may lead to speech and hearing deficits

OSMF significantly impacts quality of life in its later stages, underlining the importance of early detection and management.

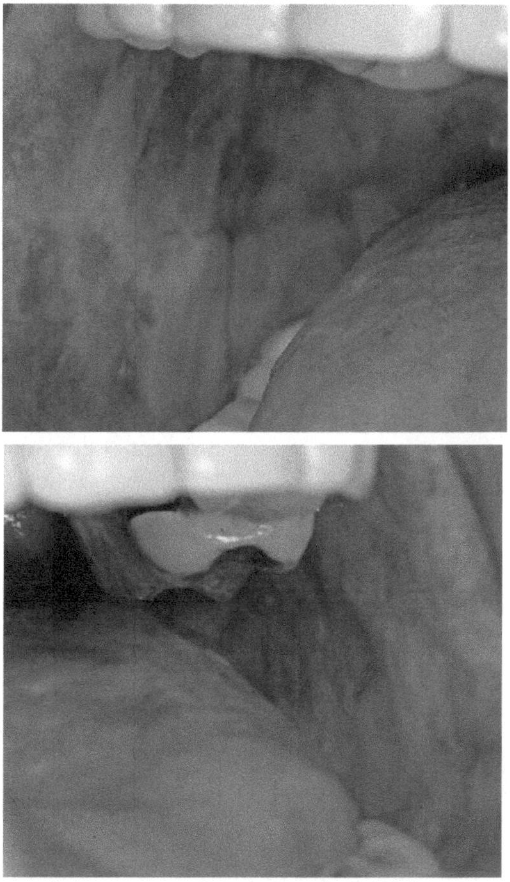

OSMF

Palatal Changes Induced by Reverse Smoking: [61]

1. **Hyperpigmentation:**
    - Well-defined diffuse or focal greyish-black pigmentation.
    - Irregular margins compared to physiological racial pigmentation.
2. **Depigmentation:**
    - Presents as pale areas in the oral mucosa surrounded by hyperpigmentation.

- Hypothesized that melanocytes act as antioxidants against tobacco toxins. Prolonged reverse smoking reduces melanin production.
- May also be described as palatal keratosis.

3. **Excrescences:**
   - 1-3mm elevated areas with central dots marking minor salivary gland orifices.
   - Initial palatal reaction in reverse smokers, historically synonymous with nicotina palatini but with higher malignant potential.
4. **Potentially Malignant Lesions:**
   - Clinically indistinguishable from leukoplakia and erythroplakia.
5. **Ulceration:**
   - 'Burn' type reaction from thermal injury, often crater-like.
   - May also represent frank carcinoma

Bharath et al. [62]separated the palatal changes induced by reverse smoking into the following: • Hyperpigmentation, in which well-defined diffuse or focal greyish black pigmentation is observed, as a result of melanocyte initiation. Typically, the margins are irregular, when compared to physiological racial pigmentation which presents as asymptomatic dark brown macules with less well defined borders.

• Depigmentation, presents as pale areas in the oral mucosa, often surrounded by areas of hyperpigmentation. Bharath et al, hypothesised that melanocytes act as an antioxidant that scavenge the toxic products produced by tobacco during combustion. Prolonged reverse smoking may deprive this melanin defense barrier causing a reduction of melanin production. Depigmentation may also be described as palatal keratosis Excrescences describe approximately 1-3mm elevated areas with central dots which mark the orifices of minor salivary gland in the palatal mucosa. These represent the initial palatal reaction in reverse smokers. Excrescences have been often historically used synonymously with nicotina palatini observed in conventional smokers, however, carry a higher malignant potential. The orifices are often referred to as central umbilications. Potentially Malignant Lesions: These areas are clinically indistinguishable from leukoplakia and erythroplakia. These conditions have been described in chapters in this series.

• Ulceration: These represent a 'burn' type reaction of the palatal mucosa from thermal injury, these ulcers are often crater-like. Ulceration may be the direct result of thermal injury, however, may also represent frank carcinoma

In addition, multimorphic lesions with all the above have been described where all or some the above palatal changes coexist in a single lesion

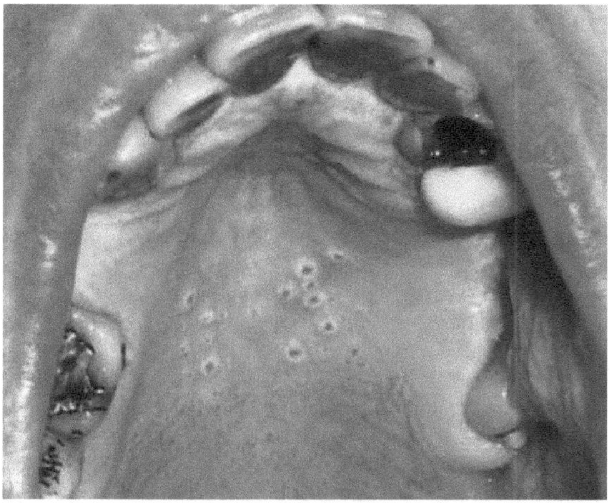

INVESTIGATION AND HISTOPATHOLOGY

Histopathological evaluation plays a crucial role in the diagnosis and assessment of oral potentially malignant disorders (OPMDs). Biopsies, obtained from suspicious lesions, are subjected to histopathological analysis to determine the presence of dysplastic changes or malignant transformation. .Histopathological examination provides valuable information about the cellular characteristics, tissue architecture, and degree of dysplasia, aiding in the diagnosis, prognosis, and treatment planning for patients with OPMDs. [63]

Non-invasive diagnostic techniques have gained attention in the evaluation of OPMDs, offering advantages such as simplicity, patient comfort, and the potential for repeated assessments. However, their diagnostic accuracy may be limited compared to histopathological evaluation. Oral brush cytology is a non-invasive technique that involves collecting cells from the surface of the oral mucosa for cytological analysis. While it provides a convenient method for initial screening, it has limitations in terms of sensitivity and specificity. Salivary biomarkers have also been investigated for their potential in OPMD detection. These biomarkers include genetic, epigenetic, and protein-based markers that can be measured in saliva samples. Optical techniques such as autofluorescence, chemiluminescence, and narrow-band imaging have shown promise in enhancing the visualization of suspicious lesions and aiding in their diagnosis.[64]

Leukoplakia requires clinicopathological correlation for a definitive diagnosis and prognosis. Oral leukoplakia (OL) is a provisional clinical diagnosis made after excluding other disorders. Although the histopathological features of OL are non-specific, the diagnosis and prognosis of OL and proliferative verrucous leukoplakia (PVL) rely on both clinical and histological features. Several adjuncts, such as tissue autofluorescence evaluation, have been proposed as visual aids for diagnosing potentially malignant disorders and malignant lesions of the oral mucosa. However, these devices should be considered clinical adjuncts rather than diagnostic tools.

The gold standard for confirming oral leukoplakia involves performing an incisional biopsy of the white patch and conducting histopathological analysis. This diagnostic biopsy is essential to confirm or refute OL and exclude other pathologies like oral squamous cell carcinoma (OSCC). The biopsy also assesses the presence and degree of epithelial dysplasia.

Histopathological findings may range from simple epithelial hyperplasia to varying degrees of dysplasia In non-homogeneous OL and extensive PVL lesions, selecting the correct site for biopsy is crucial to avoid underdiagnosis. Errors in biopsy procedures may contribute to misdiagnosis, potentially missing epithelial dysplasia or carcinoma. Therefore, multiple incisional biopsies are often necessary for comprehensive lesion mapping. Periodic mapping biopsies may be indicated in PVLs to detect different grades of dysplasia or OSCC. However, frequent biopsies can alter the disease's natural history and may increase the chances of malignancy development. Approximately 10-17% of non-homogeneous OL and PVL cases may be missed with a single biopsy.[65]

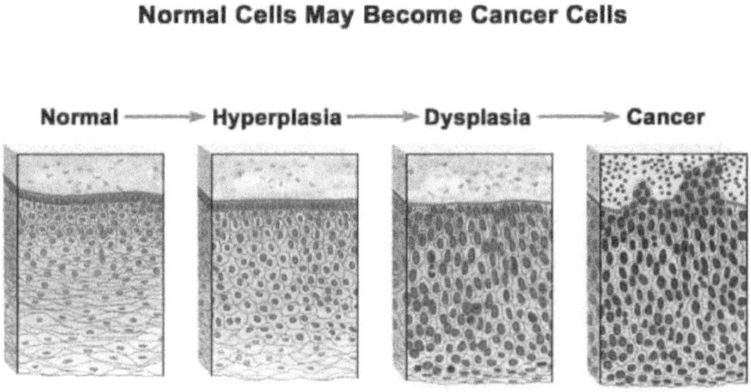

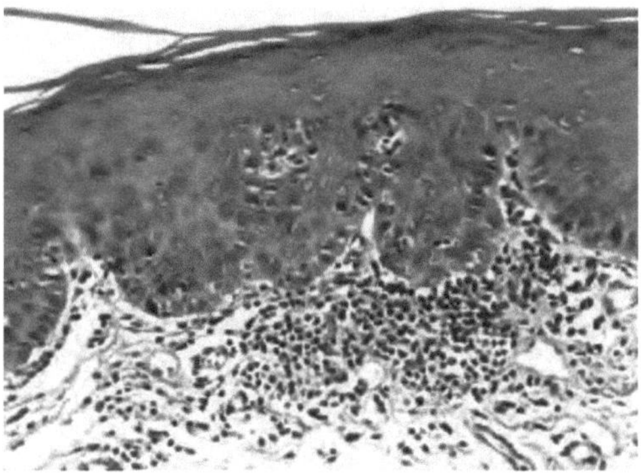

Oral epithelium with severe characteristics of dysplasia

Several adjuncts, which evaluate tissue autofluorescence, have been proposed as a visual diagnostic aid for potentially malignant disorders and malignant lesions of the oral mucosa Optical fluorescence imaging may be an adjunct to complete oral examination in clinical settings, however, these devices should be considered as clinical adjuncts and not as diagnostic tool.

The gold standard procedure to confirm the clinical diagnosis of oral leukoplakia is to perform a representative incisional biopsy of the white patch lesion and send tissue for histopathological analysis . Diagnostic biopsy is mandatory to confirm or refute the diagnosis of OL. The biopsy, and the subsequent histopathological examination, allow one to exclude other pathologies which may present as a white patch and assess for candida colonisation within the epithelium . Biopsy is necessary to exclude the diagnosis of oral squamous cell carcinoma (OSCC) and to evaluate the presence of and degree of epithelial dysplasia . Histopathological findings associated with oral leukoplakia can range from simple epithelial hyperplasia with hyperparakeratosis or hyper(ortho) keratosis, the presence or absence of and degree of epithelial dysplasia .

In order to achieve uniformity in classification and reporting, the WHO Collaborating Centre for Oral Cancer recommends the following pathology report as histopathological confirmed diagnosis of OL: 'keratosis with no / mild / moderate / severe dysplasia, consistent with oral leukoplakia'. This minimizes misclassification and assists in the subsequent management and treatment decisions.

Microscopic examination also gives the opportunity to exclude the presence of malignancy as a small area of OSCC may be clinically difficult to identify, especially in white and red patches

In non-homogeneous OL and extensive PVL lesions, it is important to select the correct site (or sites) for incisional biopsy to avoid underdiagnosis. Histopathological examination may lead to variable results within the field of the same lesion Errors during biopsy procedures, often linked to taking samples from non-representative sites, may also contribute to misdiagnosis. This common error may underestimate epithelial dysplasia or miss a diagnosis of squamous cell carcinoma. Therefore, in non-homogeneous white and red patches, multiple incisional biopsies may be indicated to achieve complete mapping of the lesion . Multiple and periodic mapping biopsies may be indicated in PVLs to detect different grades of dysplasia or OSCC. However, it must be noted that multiple and frequent biopsy may alter the natural history of the disease and interventions may significantly increase the chances of developing a malignancy. In non-homogeneous OL and PVL, approximately 10%–17% of cases may be missed by undertaking only a single biopsy

The histopathological features of PVL are not pathognomonic and are non-specific, ranging from hyperkeratosis in the early stages, to verrucous hyperplasia, and different grades of dysplasia . In addition, PVL cases characterised clinically by an inflammatory component or lichenoid appearance may show a 'lichenoid' lymphocytic band, and be misdiagnosed as OLP For this reason, the definitive diagnosis of PVL is made on the basis of a combination of clinical and histopathological findings Every white lesion, which becomes warty and exophytic, with spread over time and recurrence after treatment, should be considered as PVL.

When obtaining a biopsy from a suspected PVL lesion, as well as non-homogeneous OL, it is important to choose the most representative parts to avoid underdiagnosis Histopathological examination may lead to a variable diagnosis within the same lesion

For this reason, multiple mapping biopsies are often recommended Multiple and periodic mapping biopsies are indicated in PVL to detect different grades of dysplasia or to exclude OSCC It has been reported in PVL and non homogeneous OL that approximately 10%–17% of OSCC cases may be missed by performing only a single biopsy

Erythroplakia:

A solitary lesion with well demarcated borders aids the practitioner to clinically distinguish erythroplakia from other disorders. These solitary lesions may be discovered incidentally by the general dental practitioners prompting referral. Urgent biopsy is essential to exclude neoplastic change. The histopathological features that may be found have been described above, thin and atrophic epithelium, lack of keratin and hyperplasia. Hematoxylin and eosin is the most common staining used by histopathologists in the diagnosis of erythroplakia A recent systematic review calculated the overall risk of malignant transformation as 33.1% and a malignant transformation rate per year at 2.7%. However, there was high degree of heterogeneity amongst the studies included The malignant transformation rate is observably higher in cohorts with other known risk factors for oral cancer, such as betel quid chewing, tobacco habits, alcohol consumption and poor nutritional status. Currently, there is no reliable diagnostic tool to identify which lesions will undergo malignant transformation. Hypothesised sites that undergo the highest rate of malignant transformation include the floor of mouth and ventral tongue regions. The exact mechanism causing malignant transformation remains unknown Image cytometry DNA ploidy analysis combined with grade of dysplasia has been shown to have the highest predictive value, when considering malignant transformation and OPMDs Destructive and abhorrent patterns of intraepithelial papillary capillary loop of Narrow Band Images (NBI) have been implicated as indicators for high-grade dysplasia, carcinoma in situ and invasive carcinoma in erythroplakia. NBI is not routinely used and the application of this optical technique will remain to be seen Recently, optical techniques utilising light-based imaging, such as tissue autofluorescence and chemiluminescence have been developed to facilitate the early detection of mucosal changes indicating changes for oral cancer. Other adjuncts include oral exfoliative cytology (brush biopsies), and the use of contrast agents/vital dyes. However, the efficacy of these when used solely to differentiate between benign and potentially malignant/malignant disorders has yet to be demonstrated and conventional oral examination with biopsy remains the gold standard

Erythroplakia often demonstrates varying degrees of dysplasia and epithelial). The surface usually lacks keratinization, correlating with the red clinical appearance. The lamina propria often exhibits prominent vascularity and a chronic inflammatory infiltrate.[66]

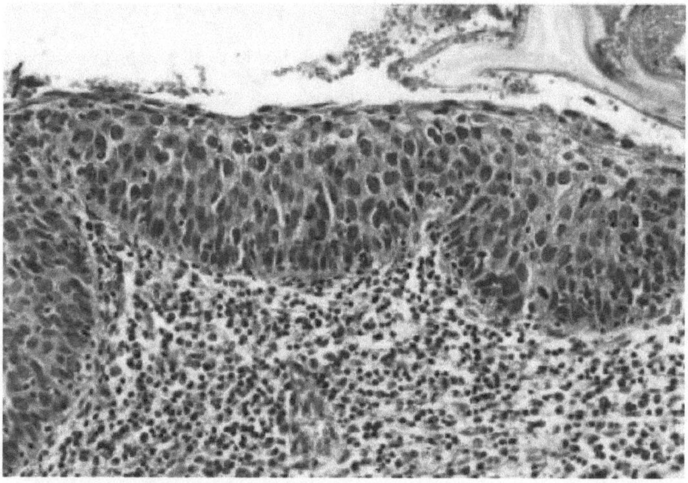

Palatal Lesions in Reverse Smokers

Careful enquiry into recreational habits and a history of long-standing reverse smoking should lead to a high degree of clinical suspicion when changes are observed in the palatal mucosa. Conventional oral examination with appropriate lighting should be sufficient to detect palatal oral mucosal changes. Gomez et al., proposed a grading system for these lesions: • Grade 0 in which no palatal changes are observed

• Grade 1 in which mild palatal changes are observed such as 'red circular areas over a slightly raised blanched mucosa of the glandular zone of the hard palate.'

• Grade 2 represent moderate palatal changes such as 'papules of 2-4mm with central umbilication less than 2mm of diameter. Moderate changes include hyperkeratinization and premalignant changes like leukoplakia.'

• Grade 3 represent severe palatal changes such as 'papules greater than 4-5mm in size with central umblicus 2-4 mm in size or characterised by crater like ulcerations surrounded by keratinization'.

• Grade 4 lesions represent palatal carcinoma Due to the malignant potential of PLRS, biopsy of these lesions is paramount and may show varying grades of dysplasia or carcinoma. Specifically, excrescences, histologically show hyperplasia of ductal epithelium

OSMF

The characteristic histological feature of oral submucous fibrosis is the presence of dense fibrosis with reduced vascularization of the lamina propria. Early lesions can be challenging to diagnose before the fibrosis is marked. Special stains, such as Van Gieson, can aid visualization of the parallel arrangement of collagen fibers marked. Hyperkeratosis and epithelial atrophy have also been reported as epithelial changes. The inflammatory infiltrate can be variable and may even show a lichenoid inflammatory pattern. Importantly, biopsies should be assessed for the presence of epithelial dysplasia, which is seen in up to 15% of cases.[67] Conventional oral examination, followed by biopsy remains the gold standard for diagnosis

MEDICAL MANAGEMENT STRATERGIES OF TOBACCO ASSOSICIATED OPMD

The prevention of OPMDs focuses on minimizing risk factors associated with the development and progression of these lesions to reduce the incidence of oral cancer.

Tobacco Cessation

Both smoking and smokeless tobacco are significant risk factors for OPMDs.

Public health interventions, counseling, nicotine replacement therapy (NRT), and behavioral support are effective.

There are two types of interventions, namely non-pharmacological and pharmacological. Non-pharmacological interventions are important as they are cost effective such as Counselling by medical practitioners, Smoking cessation strategies delivered by nurses and support organizations, Telephonic call back and follow-up, health education and heavy taxation on tobacco products. When they are combine with pharmacological interventions, give better abstinence rates, even in resistant cases with frequent relapses. Various effective pharmaco-therapeutic methods for tobacco cessation are now available and should be advised to the tobacco abusers. Pharmacotherapy should be strongly recommended to all persons with severe dependence, tobacco users with multiple failed self-attempts, tobacco users unable to abstain with brief intervention alone.

- **Approaches for tobacco cessation at the individual level may be divided into 2 types-**

1. **Non Pharmacologic intervention:-**It includes

A) **Behavioural interventions:** A variety of behaviour therapies, ranging in complexity from simple advice offered by a physician or other health care providers or much more extensive therapy offered by counsellors, have been shown to be efficacious for tobacco cessation. The Five A's (Ask, Advise, Assess, Assist and Arrange) and Five R's (Relevance, Risk, Rewards, Repetitions, Roadblocks) are five to fifteen minute research based counseling approach that has proven global success.

B) Telephone counseling: The effectiveness of telephone counseling in aiding smoking cessation has been well-documented, particularly through the protocol developed by the American Cancer Society (ACS). This protocol, implemented since 2000, has significantly increased the success rates of sustained quitting, particularly among younger smokers. Despite its success, there is room for improvement in terms of cost efficiency.

2. Pharmacologic interventions: Various effective pharmacological methods of smoking cessation are available which can help a person to quit smoking.

➢ **BROAD APPROACHES TO PHARMACOTHERAPY**

❖ **Pharmacotherapy should be strongly recommended to**

- All persons with severe dependence.
- Tobacco users with multiple failed self-attempts.
- Tobacco users unable to abstain with brief intervention alone.

- It may be suggested to all persons with lower levels of dependence who feel the need for some external help. For this group, lower doses of pharmacotherapy may be effective.

- However, it is important to note that "no form of pharmacotherapy is a substitute for motivation".

❖ **When to recommend pharmacotherapy?**

If available, it must be strongly recommended to tobacco users with severe dependence which can be determined by any of the clinical indicators below:

- Using tobacco within the first 30 minutes of waking up. or
- Using more than 20 cigarettes or *bidis* everyday or using very high doses of smokeless tobacco.
- A score of more than 6 on the Fagerstrom questionnaire.

- **The choice of pharmacotherapy would depend on**
  - Any contraindications or precautions for use.
  - The tobacco user's preference.
  - Cost of the treatment (particularly where the cost is out-of-pocket).
  - The clinicians' experience with recommending and supervising the pharmacotherapy.
  - Generally, pharmacotherapy is advised for 3 to 4 months. However, some studies suggest using pharmacotherapy for longer periods of up to six months or more

Type of treatment Rationale

✓ Nicotine replacement therapy

-Supplies the nicotine but eliminates other (harmful) chemicals in the tobacco product.

- Decreases the intensity of cravings and withdrawal symptoms, enabling people to function better while dealing with the social and psychological aspects of their dependence.
- May provide some of the effects for which the tobacco user used the particular tobacco product (e.g. the desired mood or immediate support to cope with stress).

- Evidence-based pharmacotherapies currently available for nicotine dependence include the following:

Nicotine replacement treatments

- Gums
- Patches
- Sprays
- Inhalers
- Lozenges
- Sublingual tablets
- Silver acetate

Non-nicotine replacement treatments

- Act on central brain receptors and minimize withdrawal from nicotine when the tobacco user suddenly stops use.

Non-nicotine pharmacotherapy:

- Bupropion

VARIOUS NICOTINE REPLACEMENT THERAPY PRODUCTS

1. SILVER ACETATE

Silver acetate chewing gum may be an alternative to nicotine-containing chewing gum when individuals have failed with the former product or when it is contraindicated. It demonstrated a modest benefit over placebo as a smoking deterrent in a minimal intervention and highly cost-effective treatment setting.[68]

A comparative study found no advantage from treatment with silver acetate chewing gum and only a short term advantage from treatment with nicotine chewing gum than ordinary chewing gum.[69]

2. NICOTINE GUMS

The usefulness of 2 mg nicotine chewing-gum as an aid to stop smoking was effective and implies a definite role for nicotine in cigarette dependence and withdrawal. Successful use of the gum requires careful attention to subjects' expectations and clear instructions on how to use it. Minor side effects were common but only gastric symptoms were more frequent with the active gum.[70]

A clear increase in the success rate was seen when the advice of general practitioners to stop smoking is accompanied by an offer of treatment with nicotine chewing gum. Author recommended that it would be feasible and effective for general practitioners to include the offer of nicotine gum and brief instructions on its use as part of a minimal intervention routine with all cigarette smokers.[71]Similarly, instructions and advice given by pharmacists might improve the smoking cessation rate in smokers receiving nicotine replacement therapy.[70]

Nicotine chewing gum is effective in improving the success rates in smoking cessation based on group therapy.[72] But in contrast, another author reported that the value of nicotine chewing gum, if any, can be quite small when it is used in general practice.[73]

The acute thermogenic effects of chewing gum containing different doses of nicotine and caffeine was assessed. Caffeine might be useful in preventing weight gain after smoking cessation if its thermogenic effect can be used to enhance nicotin's effect on long-term energy balance. [74]

Combination of sublingual pralidoxime and ipratropium (ProBAN) together combined with nicotine gum doubled the continuous sustained quit rate compared with nicotine replacement alone, with no adverse effects. Although not statistically significant due to the size of the study, this result suggests that it may be an effective therapy for smoking cessation, and larger studies are warranted.[75]

In an estimation of the safety and efficacy of treatment with 2 mg nicotine gum for smoking cessation in pregnant women who smoked daily, received individualized behavioural counselling, author suggested that despite not reducing smoking during pregnancy, use of nicotine gum increased birth weight and gestational age, two key parameters in predicting neonatal wellbeing.[76]

1. TRANSDERAML PATCHES

All transdermal nicotine doses significantly decreased the severity of nicotine withdrawal symptoms and significantly reduced cigarette use by patients who did not stop smoking. Compliance was excellent, and no serious systemic adverse effects were reported. Transdermal nicotine systems showed considerable promise as an aid to smoking cessation.[77,78] Patches were most effective for smokers with moderate nicotine dependence and for younger smokers specially.[79]

The use of 42 mg/day nicotine patch therapy is safe and should be considered initial therapy in the clinical setting among Smokeless Tobacco users who use ≥ 3 cans per week.[80]

Randomized trial on transdermal patch showed that Genetically, DRD2 genetic variants, related to relatively decreased dopaminergic tone in the mesocorticolimbic system were associated with increased risk for relapse to smoking following a cessation attempt.[81] Genetic variation in the dopamine pathway might provide a future basis for tailored smoking cessation therapies, but indicated that different genes influencing various components of this pathway might have different effects on response to smoking cessation pharmacotherapy.[82]

Transdermal nicotine patches used as an adjunct to brief advice and support in a general practice setting are an effective aid to long term cessation of smoking in highly dependent smokers.[83] Also, when it was used as an adjunct to low-intervention therapy, significantly reduced tobacco withdrawal symptoms and enhanced smoking cessation rates.[84] Similarly, Contingent vouchers (participants received vouchers contingent on abstinence from smoking), were more effective than transdermal nicotine patches in promoting abstinence.[85]

High-dose transdermal nicotine has the potential to substantially suppress the intake of tobacco smoke and could be a useful strategy for smoking cessation therapy or for reducing the harm caused by smoking[86,87] and it may delay post cessation weight gain for both men and women but factors that predict weight change with long-term abstinence from smoking could not be identified.[88]

Nicotine patch use in smokers who purchased the product as a non-prescription medicine from pharmacies was assessed and preliminary data on the non-prescription usage of transdermal nicotine when purchased through pharmacies was recorded. Twenty-eight per cent of respondents reported continuing smoking, although the number of cigarettes smoked was much less, than in the reported smoking history. Side effects were reported by 24% of patch users, but there was no evidence of significant safety problems.[89]

The feasibility of formulating mucoadhesive buccal nicotine patches, prepared using xanthan gum or carbopol as a mucoadhesive polymers and ethyl cellulose as a backing layer was observed in an invitro study. Author suggested that xanthan patches showed a reasonable fast initial release profile followed by controlled drug release over a 10-h period.[90]

2. NICOTINE GUMS AND PATCHES

Among the most highly nicotine dependent smokers the 4 mg gum is the most effective form of replacement therapy and in less highly dependent smokers the different preparations are comparable in their efficacy but the patch offers greater convenience and minimal need for instruction in its use.[91]

Smokers without alcohol problems showed that combination therapy (nicotine patch plus gum) was more effective than monotherapy (nicotine patch) for smoking cessation.[92]

3. NASAL NICOTINE INHALAR:

The more rapid and efficient absorption of nicotine from the nasal nicotine solution than from nicotine chewing gum suggests that it might prove a useful aid to giving up smoking. It might be particularly useful in smokers for whom the gum is less suitable on account of dentures or peptic ulcers or who experience nausea and dyspeptic symptoms from the gum.[93]Another author also suggested that Nicotine inhaler appeared safe to use and increased success rates of smoking cessation attempts. The treatment was well tolerated, and no serious adverse events were reported.[94]

In an evaluation of the efficacy and safety of nicotine 4 mg gum or nicotine 10 mg inhaler in helping smokers to reduce or quit smoking, both resulted in a significantly higher

abstinence rate than placebo. In addition a large number of smokers managed to reduce their cigarette consumption by more than 50% compared to baseline.[95]

Similarly, the efficacy of the nicotine inhaler plus nicotine patch vs nicotine inhaler plus placebo patch for smoking cessation was compared, author reported that treatment with the nicotine inhaler plus nicotine patch resulted in significantly higher cessation rates than inhaler plus placebo patch[96] whereas in other study, author found that in hospital patients, NRT given as regular daily patches plus an inhalator to be used as needed, did not add to the smoking cessation rate achieved at 1 year by regular advice and support, despite significantly increasing the cessation rate at 1 week.[96]

In a comparison to monitor the effect of a novel nicotine delivery device (Eclipse) on cigarette smoking, carbon monoxide and nicotine concentrations, and motivation to give up smoking with the smoker's own brand of cigarette and Nicotrol inhaler. Eclipse can dramatically decrease cigarette consumption without causing withdrawal symptoms or decreases in nicotine concentrations or motivation to quit altogether. Unlike the inhaler, Eclipse produces an increase in carbon monoxide concentration so it may not be a safer cigarette.[97]

4. NICOTINE SPRAY:

A trial, to assess the impact of instructional guidance in the regular use of use nicotine nasal spray (NNS) on the true use of NNS, recommended the use of NNS only when craving appeared for heavy smokers willing to quit seems acceptable compared to prescribing hourly administration. [98]

In a comparison among nicotine polacrilex (gum), a transdermal patch, nasal spray, and an inhaler, the products did not differ in their effects on withdrawal discomfort, urges to smoke, or rates of abstinence. Compliance with recommended nicotine replacement treatment use was high for the patch, low for gum, and very low for the spray and the inhaler. The spray was under used because of adverse effects more often than the other products. [99] Another study also suggested that the unpleasant side effects like nasal irritation and burning followed by complaints about the taste and smell, poor adherence, and consequent lack of efficacy observed in randomized open label trial did not support the use of nicotine nasal spray as an adjunct to counseling for adolescent smokers wishing to quit. [100]

5. NICOTINE LOZENGES:

A study tested the safety and efficacy of nicotine polacrilex (2- and 4-mg nicotine lozenges) for smoking cessation. Smokers who used more lozenges achieved significantly better treatment effects. Use of the active lozenge also resulted in reduced craving and withdrawal. Most adverse events were moderate and resembled those seen with nicotine gum. The nicotine lozenge was a safe and effective new treatment for smoking cessation in low- and high-dependence smokers.[101] Another study determined if the 4-mg nicotine lozenge with a behavioural intervention could facilitate smokeless tobacco (ST) use reduction among ST users compared with a behavioural intervention alone, author found the use of reduction strategies for ST users not interested in quitting deserves further evaluation as an intervention strategy.

In contrast, a randomized trial compared the effectiveness of transdermal nicotine vs. nicotine lozenge for smoking cessation, the author found Transdermal nicotine may be more effective than nicotine lozenge for smokers who prefer transdermal nicotine and do not smoke to alleviate emotional distress or stimulate cognitive function.[102]

PHARMACOLOGICAL STRATERGIES

The primary goal in managing Oral Potentially Malignant Disorders (OPMDs) is to monitor and prevent their progression to oral cancer. Various treatment and management strategies have been proposed to reduce this risk. The main approaches include medical treatment, which involves topical or systemic therapies; clinical observation, where no immediate intervention is taken but strict clinical and histological surveillance is maintained; and surgical intervention using techniques such as scalpel excision, laser surgery (excision and vaporization), and cryosurgery. However, there is no established consensus on the most effective approach for managing OPMDs.[102]

Pharmacological interventions play a crucial role in the management of oral leukoplakia and oral submucous fibrosis (OSMF). These therapies aim to reduce lesion size, prevent malignant transformation, and alleviate symptoms. Various classes of pharmacological agents, including antioxidants, vitamins, retinoids, and herbal formulations, have been explored for their potential chemopreventive and therapeutic effects

Antioxidants

Antioxidants play a crucial role in mitigating oxidative stress, a key factor in carcinogenesis, particularly in conditions like oral leukoplakia. By neutralizing reactive oxygen species (ROS), antioxidants prevent oxidative damage to vital biomolecules such as DNA, proteins, and lipids, thereby reducing the risk of genetic mutations and cellular dysfunction. Additionally, they inhibit lipid peroxidation, safeguarding cell membranes from structural damage and preserving cellular integrity. Antioxidants also modulate inflammatory pathways by downregulating pro-inflammatory cytokines, including tumor necrosis factor-alpha (TNF-α) and interleukin-6 (IL-6), which are known to contribute to tumor progression. Furthermore, they enhance cellular repair mechanisms by promoting DNA repair and facilitating apoptosis in damaged cells, thereby preventing malignant transformation and supporting overall cellular homeostasis. [103]

- **Lycopene**

Mechanism of action

Lycopene exerts its protective effects against oral carcinogenesis through multiple mechanisms. One of its primary functions is the scavenging of reactive oxygen species (ROS), particularly singlet oxygen and peroxyl radicals, which significantly reduces oxidative stress and prevents cellular damage. Additionally, lycopene modulates genetic pathways by downregulating pro-carcinogenic genes while enhancing tumor suppressor genes such as p53, a key regulator of cell cycle arrest and apoptosis. Another crucial mechanism involves the inhibition of the nuclear factor kappa B (NF-κB) pathway, which plays a vital role in promoting inflammation and tumor progression. By suppressing NF-κB activation, lycopene reduces the expression of inflammatory mediators such as interleukin-1 beta (IL-1β) and tumor necrosis factor-alpha (TNF-α). Furthermore, lycopene induces apoptosis in dysplastic oral epithelial cells by upregulating Bax, a pro-apoptotic protein, while downregulating Bcl-2, an anti-apoptotic protein, thus triggering programmed cell death in abnormal cells. Another critical anti-cancer property of lycopene is its ability to inhibit angiogenesis by suppressing vascular endothelial growth factor (VEGF), which restricts the blood supply necessary for the survival and proliferation of precancerous and malignant cells [104]

Tapasya Karemore et al. (2024) . [105] conducted a systematic review on lycopene's efficacy in managing oral leukoplakia, analyzing four RCTs with oral lycopene doses ranging from 4 mg to 8 mg daily over 2–3 months. The results showed significant lesion size reduction, symptom improvement, and no adverse effects, highlighting lycopene's potential as a safe and cost-effective treatment. However, limitations included a small number of RCTs, variability in study designs, and short follow-up periods, necessitating further standardized trials to confirm long-term efficacy.

Singh et al. (2004) [106] conducted a randomized, double-blind, placebo-controlled study to evaluate the efficacy of oral lycopene in treating oral leukoplakia. Fifty-eight patients were randomly assigned to receive either 8 mg/day lycopene, 4 mg/day lycopene, or a placebo for three months. The study found that lycopene supplementation resulted in significant clinical improvement in leukoplakia lesions compared to the placebo, with the 8 mg/day dosage showing greater efficacy than the 4 mg/day dosage. No significant adverse effects were reported. The authors concluded that lycopene is effective and safe for the management of oral leukoplakia, with higher doses providing better outcomes.

In their 2020 study, Gopinath et al.[107] evaluated the efficacy of combining lycopene with corticosteroids and hyaluronidase in managing Oral Submucous Fibrosis (OSMF). Lycopene was administered orally, while corticosteroids and hyaluronidase were delivered via intralesional injections. The combination therapy resulted in significant improvements, notably increased mouth opening and reduced burning sensations. However, the study faced limitations, including a small sample size, short follow-up duration, and the absence of a standardized dosage regimen. Additionally, factors such as patient adherence and variability in disease severity may have influenced the outcomes.

In their 2020 study, Saini et al.[108] investigated the efficacy of oral lycopene supplementation in managing Oral Submucous Fibrosis (OSMF). Patients receiving lycopene exhibited a significant increase in mouth opening over time, likely due to lycopene's antifibrotic properties that enhance tissue elasticity. Additionally, there was a notable reduction in burning sensations, attributed to lycopene's anti-inflammatory and mucoprotective effects. The study did not report any significant side effects, suggesting lycopene's favorable safety profile. However, limitations included a small sample size, short follow-up duration, and lack of a standardized dosage regimen. Furthermore, variations in disease severity and patient adherence may have influenced the outcomes.

There is lack of literature in management of oral erythroplakia , PVL and Palatal lesions with lycopene

Lycopene **can be considered a safe and effective adjunctive therapy** in leukoplakia and early OSMF due to its antioxidant and anti-inflammatory effects. However, its long-term efficacy in preventing **oral cancer and advanced fibrosis progression requires further high-quality, long-term clinical trials**. Until more robust data is available, lycopene should be used **as a supplementary treatment rather than a standalone therapy**.

- **Beta-carotene**

Mechanism of action

Beta-carotene, a vitamin A precursor, protects against oral potentially malignant disorders (OPMDs) and carcinogenesis through antioxidant, anti-inflammatory, and immune-modulating mechanisms. It neutralizes reactive oxygen species (ROS), preventing oxidative DNA damage and lipid peroxidation, reducing malignant transformation risk. Beta-carotene also regulates gene expression by enhancing tumor suppressor genes like p53 while downregulating pro-inflammatory cytokines such as TNF-α, IL-6, and NF-κB, which contribute to inflammation-induced carcinogenesis. Additionally, it boosts immune surveillance by activating NK cells and cytotoxic T lymphocytes, aiding in the elimination of dysplastic or malignant cells. It also supports epithelial integrity by promoting keratinocyte differentiation and reducing hyperplasia in premalignant lesions.

Toru Nagao et al.[109] conducted a randomized controlled trial evaluating the efficacy of low-dose beta-carotene (10 mg/day) combined with vitamin C (500 mg/day) in reducing oral leukoplakia lesion size. Beta-carotene was administered orally, showing significant clinical improvement with a favorable safety profile. However, the study had limitations, including a short follow-up duration, lack of data on long-term malignant transformation prevention, and potential variability in patient response. Reported side effects were minimal, though high doses of beta-carotene have been linked to carotenodermia and, in smokers, an increased risk of lung cancer. Further long-term studies are necessary to confirm its role in oral cancer prevention.

Lodi et al. (2016) [110] conducted a Cochrane systematic review assessing various interventions for oral leukoplakia, including beta-carotene. Beta-carotene was administered orally and showed potential efficacy in lesion healing. However, the study highlighted significant limitations, including high relapse rates, variability in treatment response, and insufficient long-term follow-up to determine its role in preventing malignant transformation. Reported side effects included gastrointestinal discomfort and skin discoloration (carotenodermia), though severe adverse effects were rare. The review concluded that while beta-carotene may offer short-term clinical benefits, larger, long-duration trials are necessary to establish its long-term effectiveness and safety in preventing oral cancer.

Nilesh et al. (2021) [111]demonstrated that beta-carotene, administered orally as part of a multi-drug antioxidant therapy, significantly improved mouth opening and reduced burning sensations in early-stage Oral Submucous Fibrosis (OSMF). Its antioxidant effects helped counter oxidative stress, regulate collagen metabolism, and support epithelial repair, contributing to enhanced tissue elasticity and reduced oral discomfort. However, the study had limitations, including a small sample size, short follow-up duration, and lack of standardized dosing protocols. Additionally, its effectiveness was primarily observed in early-stage OSMF, limiting its applicability in advanced cases. The findings underscore beta-carotene's potential as a preventive therapeutic option, but further large-scale, long-term studies are needed to validate its efficacy and safety.

There is lack of literature on the role of management of PVL Erythroplakia and palatal lesions with betacarotene.

While **beta-carotene may provide symptomatic relief and short-term clinical benefits**, its long-term role in preventing oral cancer and disease progression remains **uncertain**. It **can be considered as an adjunct therapy** in leukoplakia and early OSMF, but larger, long-term trials are necessary to confirm its effectiveness and safety.

- **Vitamin Therapy**

Mechanism of Action

Vitamin supplementation is considered a potential adjunct in the management of oral leukoplakia due to its ability to modulate cellular processes, enhance immune responses, and reduce oxidative stress. Vitamin therapy plays a crucial role in preventing and managing oral potentially malignant disorders (OPMDs) by modulating oxidative stress, inflammation, and cellular repair mechanisms. Various vitamins, particularly vitamin A, vitamin C, vitamin E, and vitamin D, exhibit protective effects through different pathways.

Vitamin A (Retinoids) regulate cell differentiation and proliferation by binding to nuclear retinoic acid receptors (RARs) and retinoid X receptors (RXRs), influencing gene transcription to promote normal epithelial differentiation and reduce dysplasia. Retinoids also suppress abnormal keratinization, which is a key feature of oral leukoplakia, and induce apoptosis in dysplastic cells by modulating pro-apoptotic proteins like Bax and downregulating Bcl-2, an anti-apoptotic protein

Vitamin C (Ascorbic Acid) acts as a potent antioxidant by scavenging reactive oxygen species (ROS) and reducing oxidative stress-induced DNA damage. It enhances collagen synthesis, contributing to tissue repair in conditions like oral submucous fibrosis (OSMF), and also supports immune function by enhancing natural killer (NK) cells and T-cell activity, which helps combat dysplastic cell proliferation .

Vitamin E (Tocopherols) prevents lipid peroxidation, thereby protecting cell membranes from oxidative damage. It also modulates inflammatory pathways by inhibiting nuclear factor kappa B (NF-κB), which reduces the expression of pro-inflammatory cytokines such as IL-6 and TNF-α that are associated with carcinogenesis. Additionally, tocopherols enhance immune surveillance and promote apoptosis in dysplastic epithelial cells

Vitamin D plays a crucial role in immunomodulation and cell cycle regulation. It exerts anti-proliferative and pro-apoptotic effects by regulating the vitamin D receptor (VDR) pathway. Furthermore, vitamin D suppresses angiogenesis by inhibiting vascular endothelial growth factor (VEGF), reducing the nutrient supply to dysplastic and malignant cells. It also possesses anti-fibrotic properties, making it beneficial in conditions like OSMF by reducing fibroblast proliferation and extracellular matrix deposition

Jewel Kai Lin See et al. (2023)[112] reviewed the role of vitamins A, C, D, and E in managing oral leukoplakia, highlighting their chemopreventive effects, administration methods, and limitations. Vitamin A (retinoids), typically given orally or topically in doses of 300,000–900,000 IU/day, regulates cell proliferation but is limited by severe side effects such as mucocutaneous dryness, liver toxicity, and high relapse rates. Vitamin C, administered orally at 500–1000 mg/day, acts as an antioxidant with minimal side effects, though its clinical efficacy remains inconsistent. Vitamin E, taken at 400–800 IU/day, enhances antioxidant protection but may increase bleeding risk, and its benefits in leukoplakia are variable. Vitamin D, supplemented at 1000–4000 IU/day, aids immune modulation and cell differentiation, yet evidence on its direct impact on leukoplakia is limited, and excessive intake may cause hypercalcemia and kidney dysfunction. Despite their potential, these vitamins lack standardized dosing regimens, and their long-term efficacy remains uncertain, necessitating further large-scale clinical trials to establish their role in leukoplakia management.

Islam M. et al. (2023) [113] conducted a cross-sectional study evaluating the preventive effects of vitamins A, C, and E in patients with oral leukoplakia over different time intervals. The study reported that 11.63% of patients showed complete lesion improvement after 24 weeks, indicating a potential chemopreventive role for these vitamins. Vitamin A, known for its role in cell differentiation, was administered primarily in oral form, while vitamins C and E, acting as antioxidants, were given orally to reduce oxidative stress. Despite these promising results, the study faced limitations such as a lack of a control group, variability in patient adherence, and the need for longer follow-up to assess the durability of the treatment response. Additionally, potential side effects, including hypervitaminosis A, gastrointestinal discomfort, and bleeding tendencies with high-dose vitamin E, were not extensively analyzed. Further well-designed, large-scale clinical trials are required to confirm these findings and establish standardized treatment protocols for the chemoprevention of leukoplakia.

Sune et al. (2024)[114] reviewed the role of oxidative stress in Oral Submucous Fibrosis (OSMF) and the therapeutic potential of antioxidant vitamins A, C, and E in its management. The study found that patients who received these vitamins experienced symptomatic improvements, including reduced burning sensations and enhanced tissue flexibility. Vitamin A, known for its role in epithelial repair, was administered orally, while vitamins C and E, acting as antioxidants, helped neutralize oxidative stress and support collagen modulation. However, the study had limitations, including a lack of standardized dosing, variability in patient response, and the absence of long-term follow-up to assess disease progression. Potential side effects, such as hypervitaminosis A, gastrointestinal discomfort from vitamin C, and bleeding risks associated with high-dose vitamin E, were not extensively analyzed. While the findings highlight the potential benefits of antioxidant therapy in OSMF, further large-scale randomized controlled trials are needed to establish definitive treatment guidelines and assess long-term efficacy.

Nallapu et al. (2015)[115] investigated the role of vitamin E as an adjunct to corticosteroid and hyaluronidase therapy in the management of Oral Submucous Fibrosis (OSMF). The study found that patients who received vitamin E supplementation alongside standard treatment showed significant improvements in mouth opening and mucosal health. Vitamin E, known for its antioxidant and mucoprotective properties, was administered orally to help reduce oxidative stress and enhance tissue healing. However, the study had limitations, including a small sample size, lack of long-term follow-up, and variability in patient response. Additionally, potential side effects, such as bleeding tendencies at higher doses, were not extensively addressed. While the findings suggest that vitamin E may enhance treatment outcomes in OSMF, further randomized controlled trials are needed to confirm its efficacy and establish optimal dosing guidelines.

Hu, Y., Wang et al. (2019) [116] studied the efficacy of systemic and topical retinoids in the management of oral leukoplakia, demonstrating their ability to reduce lesion size and reverse dysplasia. Retinoids, derived from vitamin A, were administered both orally and as topical applications, showing promising results in modulating cell differentiation and inhibiting malignant progression. However, the study highlighted significant limitations, including high recurrence rates after treatment cessation and adverse effects such as mucocutaneous dryness, cheilitis, and hepatotoxicity with long-term systemic use. Additionally, patient adherence was a challenge due to these side effects. The authors emphasized the need for further research to optimize retinoid formulations, minimize toxicity, and explore combination therapies that could enhance efficacy while reducing recurrence rates.

Rafael Poveda-Roda et al. (2010)[117] evaluated the effects of retinoids on proliferative verrucous leukoplakia (PVL) in a small patient cohort, finding that retinoid therapy contributed to a reduction in lesion size and severity. Some patients experienced lesion regression and decreased dysplasia, highlighting the potential of retinoids in managing PVL. Administered either systemically or topically, retinoids function by modulating cell differentiation and inhibiting malignant transformation. However, the study faced significant limitations, including a small sample size, lack of long-term follow-up, and variability in patient response. Additionally, adverse effects such as mucocutaneous dryness and gastrointestinal discomfort were concerns that could impact patient compliance. Due to these limitations, larger studies are needed to confirm the effectiveness of retinoids and establish standardized treatment protocols for PVL management.

For **oral leukoplakia, vitamin A (retinoids)** is the most effective, with doses ranging from **300,000–900,000 IU/day** systemically or **0.1%–0.4% retinoic acid gel** topically. It helps in reducing lesion size and reversing dysplasia, but high relapse rates and adverse effects like mucocutaneous dryness and hepatotoxicity limit its long-term use. As safer alternatives, **vitamin C (500–1000 mg/day)** and **vitamin E (400–800 IU/day)** may provide antioxidant benefits with fewer side effects.

For **oral submucous fibrosis (OSMF), vitamin E (400–800 IU/day)** is beneficial due to its mucoprotective and antifibrotic effects, particularly when used alongside corticosteroids and hyaluronidase. **Vitamin C (500–1000 mg/day)** can be used as adjunct therapy to reduce oxidative stress and improve tissue healing. However, limitations include potential bleeding risks with high-dose vitamin E and a lack of standardized treatment protocols.

For **proliferative verrucous leukoplakia (PVL), vitamin A (retinoids) 300,000–900,000 IU/day** remains the preferred option due to its ability to reduce lesion severity and dysplasia. However, recurrence rates remain high, and side effects such as mucocutaneous dryness and gastrointestinal discomfort can impact patient compliance. **Combination therapy with vitamins C and E** may improve treatment outcomes while minimizing adverse effects. Further **large-scale clinical trials** are needed to establish long-term efficacy and optimal dosing strategies.

However there is lack of literature on management of Erythroplakia, Palatal lesions with vitamin therapy.

Spirulina

Mechanism of Action

Spirulina, a blue-green microalga rich in antioxidants, vitamins, and phycocyanins, has gained attention for its potential therapeutic benefits in oral potentially malignant disorders (OPMDs), particularly oral leukoplakia. **Spirulina aids in the management of oral potentially malignant disorders (OPMDs) through its antioxidant, anti-inflammatory, and immunomodulatory properties. Rich in phycocyanin and β-carotene, it reduces oxidative stress and DNA damage while inhibiting NF-κB and pro-inflammatory cytokines (IL-6, TNF-α, COX-2) to prevent chronic inflammation. It enhances immune response by stimulating NK cells, macrophages, and T-lymphocytes, promoting dysplastic lesion regression. Additionally, spirulina induces apoptosis, inhibits cell proliferation via p53 and Bax/Bcl-2 pathways, detoxifies carcinogens, and suppresses angiogenesis, limiting lesion progression.**

These combined effects make spirulina a promising natural adjunct in preventing malignant transformation of OPMDs

Kulkarni et al. (2024)[118] conducted a systematic review assessing the efficacy of **spirulina** in the management of **oral potentially malignant disorders (OPMDs)**, analyzing five clinical trials with varying **dosages and treatment durations**. While some studies reported a **significant reduction in lesion size and severity**, others found **minimal or no improvement**, highlighting **inconsistencies in treatment response**. Variability in **dosing regimens, study design, and sample sizes**, along with **short follow-up durations**, contributed to these mixed results. Additionally, the review identified a **high risk of bias**, including **lack of randomization and placebo control** in several studies, limiting the reliability of conclusions. Despite its **antioxidant and anti-inflammatory properties**, the definitive role of spirulina in **OPMD management remains unclear**, and **well-designed randomized controlled trials (RCTs)** with standardized dosing protocols are necessary to establish its efficacy.

Koothati Ramesh Kumar et al. (2022)[119] conducted a comparative study evaluating the efficacy of **spirulina and green tea extract** in managing **oral leukoplakia**, with both treatments administered **orally**. The results indicated that **spirulina demonstrated superior efficacy** in reducing **lesion size and improving clinical and histopathological outcomes** compared to green tea extract. Both interventions were **well-tolerated**, with **no significant adverse effects reported**, reinforcing their potential as **safe, natural therapeutic options**. However, **limitations** included **variability in treatment duration, small sample size, and lack of long-term follow-up**, necessitating **larger, well-controlled trials** to confirm their role in **oral leukoplakia management** and establish **standardized dosing protocols**.

No research has been identified regarding the role of spirulina in management of erythroplakia PVL and palatal lesions in reverse smokers.

Spirulina shows promise in managing **oral leukoplakia and OSMF** due to its **antioxidant and anti-inflammatory properties**, with studies reporting **lesion size reduction and clinical improvement**. However, **inconsistencies in results, study limitations, and lack of standardized dosing** hinder definitive conclusions. While **generally well-tolerated**, further **high-quality RCTs** are needed to confirm its efficacy and long-term benefits.

Aloe Vera

Mechanism of Action

Aloe vera, a succulent plant with well-documented medicinal properties, has been explored as a potential therapeutic agent in oral submucous fibrosis (OSMF) due to its anti-inflammatory, antioxidant, wound-healing, and immunomodulatory effects.

Gopinath et al. (2020) [120] analyzed aloe vera's effectiveness in OSMF management, reporting moderate benefits when used in combination with other treatments such as corticosteroids, physiotherapy, and hyaluronidase therapy. Patients received **oral aloe vera supplementation** and **topical application of aloe vera gel** to affected oral tissues The study found that aloe vera improved symptoms like burning sensation, fibrosis, and restricted mouth opening, though the degree of improvement varied among patients. While aloe vera has shown promise, further randomized controlled trials (RCTs) with larger sample sizes and standardized dosages are required to establish its definitive role in OSMF treatment.

No research has been identified in relation to the role of aloe vera in management of oral leukoplakia, PVL and palatal lesions in reverse smokers

Aloe vera, in both **oral and topical forms**, shows potential as an adjunctive treatment for OSMF by reducing burning sensation, fibrosis, and restricted mouth opening. While it provides **moderate benefits**, the efficacy varies among patients, necessitating **larger RCTs with standardized dosages** to confirm its role in treatment.

GARLIC EXTRACTS

Mechanism of Action

Aged garlic extract (AGE) exerts its effects in OSMF through its **antioxidant, anti-inflammatory, and antifibrotic properties**, reducing **oxidative stress, inflammation, and fibrosis**, leading to symptomatic relief.

In the study by **Kataria et al. (2023)** [121]**, aged garlic extract (AGE) was administered orally** for the management of **Oral Submucous Fibrosis (OSMF)**. Patients received **oral supplementation of AGE** due to its **antioxidant, anti-inflammatory, and antifibrotic properties**, which helped reduce oxidative stress, inflammation, and fibrosis, leading to symptomatic relief.

However, some **side effects** were reported, including **gastrointestinal discomfort (such as bloating, nausea, and acid reflux)** and **allergic reactions (skin rashes, itching, and mild respiratory issues)** in sensitive individuals. The study emphasized the **need for careful dosage optimization** and **further clinical trials** to establish the most effective and safe regimen for long-term use in OSMF treatment.

No research has been identified regarding the role of garlic extracts in management of oral leukoplakia, erythroplakia, PVL and palatal lesions in reverse smokers

AGE shows **potential benefits** in OSMF management, but reported **side effects** like gastrointestinal discomfort and allergic reactions highlight the need for **careful dosage optimization and further clinical trials** to establish its safety and efficacy.

Antiprotease Agents

Mechanism Of Action

Antiprotease agents work by inhibiting proteolytic enzymes that contribute to tissue degradation and cancer progression. **Antiprotease agents** are compounds that **inhibit proteolytic enzymes** responsible for **tissue degradation, inflammation, and tumor progression**. These agents play a crucial role in **maintaining tissue integrity** by preventing excessive breakdown of **extracellular matrix (ECM)** proteins. Proteases such as **matrix metalloproteinases (MMPs), serine proteases, and cysteine proteases** contribute to **oral carcinogenesis** by facilitating **tumor invasion, angiogenesis, and metastasis**. One of the most studied **antiprotease agents** in **oral leukoplakia** is **Bowman-Birk Inhibitor Concentrate (BBIC)**, a soybean-derived **serine protease inhibitor** known for its ability to **suppress tumorigenesis and prevent ECM degradation**.

In the **randomized, placebo-controlled trial by Armstrong WB et al. (2013) 1**[22], **Bowman-Birk Inhibitor Concentrate (BBIC) was administered orally**. The study found that the **BBIC group exhibited a 20.6% reduction in lesion size**, compared to **17.1% in the placebo group**, but this difference was **not statistically significant.Limitations** of the study included the **lack of a significant therapeutic effect when used alone**, the **small sample size**, and the **short follow-up duration**, which may have affected the results. Additionally, **BBIC's potential chemopreventive role may be more effective when combined with other agents**, rather than as a standalone treatment. **Further research with optimized dosing strategies and combination therapies** is needed to determine its efficacy in managing **oral leukoplakia**.

The systematic review by Lodi et al. (2002)[123] assessed multiple interventions for oral leukoplakia, including antiprotease agents such as Bowman-Birk Inhibitor Concentrate (BBIC). The study found no conclusive evidence supporting the efficacy of BBIC in preventing malignant transformation. Dosage limitations were noted due to a lack of standardized protocols, making it difficult to determine an optimal therapeutic regimen. Additionally, variability in treatment response, small sample sizes, and insufficient long-term follow-up restricted the reliability of the findings. While BBIC showed some potential in reducing lesion size, the results were not statistically significant, indicating that it may require combination therapy with other chemopreventive agents for meaningful clinical outcomes. Further well-structured randomized controlled trials are necessary to establish its efficacy and safety in leukoplakia management.

BBIC has shown limited efficacy in reducing oral leukoplakia lesion size, with no statistically significant results as a standalone treatment. Its potential may be enhanced in combination therapy, but further research is needed to establish its clinical utility and optimal dosing.

No research has been identified regarding the role of antiprotease agents in management of OSMF, Erythroplakia, PVL and palatal lesions in reverse smokers.

BBIC has shown **limited efficacy** in reducing oral leukoplakia lesion size, with **no statistically significant benefits** as a standalone treatment. Its **potential may be enhanced in combination therapy**, but further **well-structured trials** are needed to determine its clinical utility and optimal dosing.

Antiproliferative Agents

Mechanism of Action

Antiproliferative agents play a **crucial role in preventing the progression of OPMDs to oral cancer** by targeting **cell cycle regulation, growth factor signaling, and apoptotic pathways**. These agents work by **inhibiting dysregulated cellular**

proliferation, **blocking oncogenic pathways**, and **inducing apoptosis in abnormal epithelial cells.**

Nabil F. Saba et al. (2014) [124]conducted a clinical trial evaluating the combination of erlotinib (an epidermal growth factor receptor [EGFR] inhibitor) and celecoxib (a cyclooxygenase-2 [COX-2] inhibitor) in patients with advanced oral premalignant lesions. The study reported:A 63% histologic response rate, indicating significant reduction in dysplasia and abnormal cell proliferation.A 43% complete response, meaning a substantial number of patients showed complete regression of lesions The findings suggest that EGFR and COX-2 inhibitors have a synergistic effect, making them promising agents for chemoprevention. However, the study emphasized the need for larger trials to validate these results.

No research has been identified in relation to role of antiproliferative agents in the management of oral leukoplakia, erythroplakia, PVL and palatal lesions in reverse smokers.

The combination of **erlotinib (EGFR inhibitor) and celecoxib (COX-2 inhibitor)** shows **promising chemopreventive potential** by significantly reducing dysplasia and abnormal cell proliferation. While this approach has **not been specifically studied for OSMF**, its **synergistic effect** suggests possible therapeutic benefits, warranting **further research** to explore its efficacy in OSMF management.

- **Curcumin and Herbal Formulations**

Mechanism of Action

Curcumin, a bioactive compound derived from turmeric, has demonstrated anti-inflammatory, antioxidant, and antiproliferative properties, making it a potential therapeutic agent in oral leukoplakia and other oral potentially malignant disorders (OPMDs). Curcumin exerts its effects through multiple mechanisms, including inhibition of nuclear factor kappa B (NF-κB), which plays a central role in inflammation and carcinogenesis. By downregulating NF-κB, curcumin reduces the production of pro-inflammatory cytokines such as tumor necrosis factor-alpha (TNF-α) and interleukin-6 (IL-6), thereby limiting chronic inflammation that contributes to oral carcinogenesis. Additionally, curcumin acts as a potent antioxidant by scavenging reactive oxygen species (ROS), preventing oxidative DNA damage and lipid peroxidation. It also modulates apoptotic pathways by upregulating pro-apoptotic proteins like Bax while downregulating anti-apoptotic proteins like Bcl-2, promoting the selective elimination of dysplastic cells. Furthermore, curcumin inhibits angiogenesis by suppressing vascular endothelial growth factor (VEGF), thereby restricting blood supply to precancerous and malignant lesions.

The **Phase IIB trial by Moni Abraham Kuriakose et al. (2016)**[124] demonstrated that **curcumin supplementation effectively reduced lesion size and dysplastic changes** in oral leukoplakia patients, highlighting its **potential as a chemopreventive agent**. Curcumin was administered **orally**, showing **minimal side effects** and a **favorable safety profile**. However, **limitations** included **uncertainty in the optimal dosage**, **short follow-up duration**, and the **need for long-term studies** to confirm its role in preventing malignant transformation. Further **well-structured clinical trials** are required to establish **standardized dosing regimens** and assess its sustained efficacy

N. Vijayalaxmi et al. [126] evaluated the efficacy of curcumin oral gel in treating palatal lesions in reverse smokers. The study included two groups: **Group A**, which used curcumin oral gel on an acrylic palatal plate, and **Group B**, which received smoking cessation counseling only. Results indicated significant clinical improvement in lesion size and severity among the curcumin-treated group (**$p < 0.001$**), although cytological improvement, observed as a transition from moderate to mild dysplasia, was not statistically significant (**$p = 0.28$**). These findings suggest that curcumin has therapeutic potential for palatal lesions in reverse smokers due to its molecular targeting properties. However, smoking cessation remains critical for long-term management and prevention of disease progression.

She & Xu (2024) conducted a **comprehensive review** of studies on curcumin's role in **preventing and treating Oral Submucous Fibrosis (OSMF)**, analyzing its clinical efficacy and therapeutic potential. The **methodology** involved evaluating **preclinical and clinical trials**, focusing on curcumin's effects on **symptom relief, fibrosis regression, and inflammatory markers**. However, the review had several **limitations**, including **variability in dosages, formulations, and treatment durations** across studies, making it difficult to standardize findings. A major challenge highlighted was curcumin's **poor bioavailability**, which limits its systemic absorption and therapeutic impact, necessitating the use of **enhanced delivery systems** such as nanoparticles or liposomal formulations. Additionally, the review noted a **lack of large-scale, long-term clinical trials**, restricting definitive conclusions on its sustained benefits and potential side effects. Future research should focus on **optimizing curcumin formulations** and conducting **well-controlled randomized trials** to establish its efficacy in OSMF treatment.[127]

There is lack in literature regarding in management of Erythroplakia and PVL with Curcumin

Curcumin demonstrates potential in the management of **oral leukoplakia and OSMF** due to its **anti-inflammatory and chemopreventive properties**. However, **poor bioavailability and lack of standardized dosing** limit its widespread use. While it can be considered as an **adjunct therapy**, further **large-scale, long-term trials** are necessary to confirm its efficacy and optimal dosage.

ANTI INFLAMMATORY DRUGS

PENTOXIFYLLINE

Mechanism Of Action

Pentoxifylline (PTX), a methylxanthine derivative, has gained attention for its potential role in the treatment of oral submucous fibrosis (OSMF)—a chronic, progressive, and debilitating precancerous condition. PTX is primarily used for its hemorheologic, anti-inflammatory, and antifibrotic properties, making it a valuable adjunct therapy in improving mouth opening and alleviating symptoms in OSMF patients.

Liu, J., Chen [128] – Evaluation of PTX in OSMF Patients Conducted a randomized controlled trial (RCT) to assess pentoxifylline's effectiveness in treating OSMF. Patients were divided into two groups: Group A: Received pentoxifylline (400 mg, three times daily) alongside corticosteroids. Group B: Received only corticosteroids. Results: Significant improvement in mouth opening in the PTX-treated group. Reduced burning sensation and pain compared to corticosteroid-only therapy. Better softening of fibrotic bands, suggesting pentoxifylline's role in reversing

fibrosis. Sadaksharam et al. (2017) [96–] Combination Therapy of PTX and Corticosteroids Investigated the effects of pentoxifylline in combination with corticosteroids in OSMF patients. PTX enhanced microcirculation and improved blood flow, leading to better oxygenation of fibrotic tissues. Patients experienced faster symptomatic relief, especially in pain and stiffness. Histopathological analysis suggested partial reversal of fibrosis, though long-term effects were inconclusive. No significant adverse effects were reported, making PTX a safe and well-tolerated treatment option.

Chen X, Xie H, [129] Pentoxifylline, administered **orally**, has shown **symptomatic relief** in OSMF by improving **vascularity and reducing fibrosis**. However, **optimal dosage remains unclear**, with studies using **400 mg twice or thrice daily** showing variable efficacy. **Limitations** include **gastrointestinal discomfort, dizziness, hypotension, and bleeding risks**, restricting its widespread use. While **some clinical benefits** have been observed, **long-term efficacy and safety** require further **well-controlled trials** to establish standardized treatment protocols.

There is lack in literature regarding the role of pentoxifylline in management of Oral leukoplakia , Erythroplakia PVL and palatal lesions.

Pentoxifylline (PTX), when combined with corticosteroids, has shown significant improvement in mouth opening, pain relief, and fibrosis reduction in OSMF patients by enhancing microcirculation and tissue oxygenation. While it appears to be safe and well-tolerated, limitations such as gastrointestinal discomfort and unclear optimal dosage highlight the need for further well-controlled trials to establish its long-term efficacy and standardized treatment protocols.

Colchicine

Mechanism Of Action

Colchicine, a plant-derived alkaloid extracted from *Colchicum autumnale* (autumn crocus), has been explored as a potential therapeutic agent for OSMF due to its anti-inflammatory, antifibrotic, and immunomodulatory properties. It primarily functions by inhibiting microtubule polymerization, which affects multiple cellular pathways involved in fibrosis and inflammation.

Chen et al. (2023) [130] Colchicine shows promise in **managing OSMF** by **reducing fibroblast proliferation, collagen deposition, and inflammation**, leading to **symptomatic relief** such as **improved mouth opening and reduced burning sensation**. However, its **limitations** include **uncertain optimal dosage, short follow-up duration, and inconsistent patient response**. Reported **side effects**, including **gastrointestinal distress, hepatotoxicity, and myelosuppression**, raise concerns about its **long-term safety**. While colchicine may help **counteract fibrosis progression**, further **well-structured clinical trials** are needed to confirm its **standardized dosage, sustained efficacy, and safety profile** in OSMF treatment.

There is lack in literature regarding the role of colchine in management of Oral Leukoplakia , Erythroplakia ,PVL , Palatal lesions.

Colchicine shows **potential in OSMF management** by reducing **fibroblast proliferation, collagen deposition, and inflammation**, leading to **symptomatic relief**. However, concerns about **optimal dosage, inconsistent response, and side effects** like **gastrointestinal distress and hepatotoxicity** necessitate **further clinical trials** to establish its safety and long-term efficacy.

Placental Extract

Mechanism OF Action

Placental extract has gained attention as a biologically active therapy in treating oral submucous fibrosis (OSMF) due to its anti-inflammatory, antifibrotic, and regenerative properties. It contains growth factors, cytokines, and bioactive peptides that promote wound healing, collagen remodeling, and tissue regeneration.

Shah (2017) [131] – Comparative Study of Placental Extract and Corticosteroids Objective: To compare the efficacy of placental extract with corticosteroid therapy in improving symptoms of OSMF. Patients were divided into two groups: Group A: Received intralesional placental extract injections. Group B: Received intralesional corticosteroids. Both groups showed symptomatic relief in burning sensation, pain, and mouth opening. The placental extract group showed comparable improvements to corticosteroids but had better tissue healing and fewer side effects. Patients reported improved mucosal elasticity and relief from fibrosis-induced stiffness.

Patil et al. (2018) [132]Conducted a prospective clinical trial to evaluate placental extract therapy versus corticosteroid therapy. Results: Significant improvement in mouth opening in the placental extract group. Reduction in burning sensation and pain similar to corticosteroids. Enhanced tissue regeneration due to the growth factors present in placental extract.No major adverse effects, whereas corticosteroids were associated with localized atrophy and mild discomfort. Placental extract is a viable alternative to corticosteroids in OSMF management, offering similar or superior efficacy with fewer side effects.

There is Lack in literature regarding the role of placental extracts in management of Oral Leukoplakia, PVL Erythroplakia and palatal lesions.

Placental extract is a **promising alternative to corticosteroids** in OSMF management, offering **comparable symptomatic relief** in **burning sensation, pain, and mouth opening**, while promoting **better tissue healing and regeneration** with **fewer side effects**. Its **growth factor-rich composition** enhances mucosal elasticity, making it a **safe and effective treatment option** for OSMF.

ENZYMES

- **Collagenase**

Mechanism Of Action

Collagenase, an enzyme that breaks down collagen, has been investigated for its potential to reduce fibrosis and improve mouth opening in patients with oral submucous fibrosis (OSMF). Since OSMF is characterized by excessive collagen deposition and progressive fibrosis, collagenase therapy offers a biological approach to reversing these pathological changes.

Lin et al [133]. Conducted a clinical study evaluating the effects of collagenase injections on mouth opening and fibrosis severity in OSMF patients.Patients receiving collagenase therapy showed significant improvement in mouth opening compared to controls.Histological analysis revealed a reduction in dense collagen bundles, indicating enzymatic degradation of excess collagen.No severe adverse effects were reported, suggesting that collagenase is well-tolerated. Collagenase therapy appears to be a promising intervention for OSMF, particularly in patients with moderate to severe fibrosis.

There is Lack in literature regarding the role of collagenase in management of Leukoplaakia , Erythroplakia PVL and palatal lesions.

Collagenase therapy shows **promise in managing OSMF** by **breaking down excess collagen**, leading to **improved mouth opening and reduced fibrosis**. With **no severe adverse effects reported**, it appears to be a **well-tolerated and effective option**, but further research is needed to confirm its **long-term efficacy and standardized dosing**.

Immunomodulatory Agents

Immunomodulatory agents have been considered for PVL treatment due to their potential in modifying disease progression.

Mechanism of Action

Sirolimus, an **mTOR inhibitor**, suppresses **cell proliferation and immune activation**, reducing lesion progression in PVL. Imiquimod, a **TLR7 agonist**, enhances **innate immune response**, promoting **antiviral and antitumor effects**, leading to lesion regression. Both agents **modulate immune pathways**, but their efficacy and safety require further research.

Konrad Staines et al. (2023) [134] discussed the use of **sirolimus** as an immunomodulatory agent for PVL management, typically administered at **1–2 mg per day**, with dosage adjustments based on therapeutic drug monitoring. While sirolimus showed some potential in reducing lesion progression, studies had small sample sizes, and recurrence rates remained high, often necessitating additional surgical intervention.However, the use of sirolimus is associated with several side effects, including **mucositis, delayed wound healing, thrombocytopenia, hyperlipidemia, and an increased risk of infections**. Given these limitations, further large-scale research is needed to determine its long-term efficacy, safety, and optimal dosing regimen for PVL treatment.

Townsend et al. [135] reported a case study in which **topical imiquimod**, a **toll-like receptor 7 (TLR7) agonist**, was used to treat a **53-year-old male with recurrent proliferative verrucous leukoplakia (PVL)**. The patient had a history of multiple surgical excisions, but the lesion continued to recur. Imiquimod, an immune response modifier with antiviral and antitumor properties, was applied **topically as a 5% cream** several times per week, leading to **complete clinical and histological resolution** of the lesion. This case highlights the potential of imiquimod as a **non-surgical therapeutic option** for PVL cases that are resistant to conventional surgical treatment. However, the use of imiquimod is associated with **local and systemic side effects**, including **erythema, edema, ulceration, pain at the application site, flu-like symptoms, and fatigue**. Additionally, while this single case showed promising results, **more extensive studies are required** to determine its long-term efficacy, ideal dosing regimen, and potential for widespread use in PVL management.

There is Lack in literature regarding its role in management of Erythroplakia, Oral Leukoplakia OSMF and palatal lesions.

Sirolimus shows **some potential** in **reducing PVL lesion progression**, but its **high recurrence rates and significant side effects** necessitate **further large-scale research** to establish its long-term efficacy and optimal dosing. Imiquimod, as a **topical immune response modifier**, demonstrated **complete lesion resolution in a single case**, suggesting its **potential as a non-surgical alternative**, but **more studies** are needed to confirm its effectiveness and safety in broader PVL management.

- **LEVIMASOLE**

Mechanism Of Action

Levamisole acts as an **immunomodulator**, enhancing **T-cell function and macrophage activity**, which helps regulate **inflammatory responses** in OSMF. It also has **anti-fibrotic effects**, reducing **collagen deposition** and improving **vascular function**, leading to **symptomatic relief** and improved **mouth opening**.

Shinge et al. (2019) [136] highlights the potential efficacy of systemic levamisole (50 mg three times daily) in managing oral submucous fibrosis (OSMF) when compared to antioxidant therapy. While levamisole demonstrated symptomatic improvement, particularly in reducing burning sensation and enhancing mouth opening, its dose-dependent limitations must be considered. Prolonged use has been associated with adverse effects such as gastrointestinal discomfort, leukopenia, and vasculitis, necessitating careful monitoring. Furthermore, the results suggest that while levamisole offers a promising therapeutic option, its long-term efficacy and safety require further validation through larger, multi-center trials to establish standardized treatment regimens.

There is lack in literature regarding its role in management of Oral Leukoplakia, Erythroplakia, PVL and palatal lesions.

Levamisole shows **potential in OSMF management** by improving **burning sensation and mouth opening**, but its **dose-dependent adverse effects** like **gastrointestinal discomfort and leukopenia** require **careful monitoring**. Further **large-scale studies** are needed to confirm its **long-term efficacy and safety**.

- **Interferon Gamma**

Mechanism of Action

Interferon gamma (IFN-γ), a cytokine primarily produced by T cells and natural killer (NK) cells, has been explored for its immunomodulatory and antifibrotic properties in managing oral submucous fibrosis (OSMF). It plays a crucial role in regulating immune responses, reducing fibrosis, and inhibiting pro-fibrotic cytokines, making it a promising therapeutic option.

Shen et al. (2020) [137] Conducted a **systematic review** on IFN-γ's role in **immune modulation and fibrosis reduction**. IFN-γ **suppresses fibroblast proliferation**, reducing **excessive collagen deposition**, a hallmark of OSMF. **Downregulates pro-fibrotic cytokines** such as **TGF-β1, IL-6, and PDGF**, thereby **inhibiting fibrosis progression**.Enhances **matrix metalloproteinase (MMP) activity**, which helps degrade excessive extracellular matrix (ECM) components.Modulates the immune response by promoting **Th1 cytokine production**, shifting the balance away from a **fibrosis-inducing Th2 response**.

Rao et al. (2017)[138] the effectiveness of **intralesional IFN-γ injections** in treating **moderate to severe OSMF cases**. Patients received **50 µg of IFN-γ intralesionally twice weekly for 8 weeks**.Evaluated **mouth opening, burning sensation, and histopathological changes** before and after treatment.Significant **improvement in**

mouth opening and reduction in **burning sensation** compared to baseline ($p < 0.001$).**Histological examination showed reduced collagen deposition**, indicating **fibrosis reversal. Well-tolerated**, with **no major systemic side effects** .IFN-γ therapy appears to be an **effective and safe** alternative for OSMF, but **long-term studies are needed .**

There is lack of evidence in management of leukoplakia , erythroplakia and palatal lesions with Immunomodulatory drugs.

IFN-γ shows **promise in OSMF management** by **reducing fibrosis, suppressing fibroblast proliferation, and modulating immune responses**, leading to **improved mouth opening and symptom relief.** Intralesional IFN-γ is **well-tolerated,** but **long-term studies** are needed to confirm its **sustained efficacy and safety**.

ANTINEOPLASTIC DRUGS

- **BLEOMYCIN**

Mechanism OF Action

Bleomycin, a chemotherapeutic agent originally used for treating various cancers, has gained attention for its **potential role in managing oral leukoplakia**, a premalignant condition with the potential to progress to oral cancer. Its **cytotoxic and antiproliferative properties** make it a candidate for targeting **dysplastic epithelial cells**, reducing lesion size, and preventing malignant transformation.

Shishir Ram Shetty et al. (2016) [139] investigated the efficacy of **topical bleomycin** in treating **oral leukoplakia lesions**. The study reported: A **significant reduction in lesion size and severity**, indicating **effective cytotoxic action against dysplastic cells. Well-tolerated administration**, with most patients experiencing **minimal side effects**. However, concerns about **systemic toxicity and local adverse reactions** necessitate **careful monitoring** and **dose optimization**. The study emphasized the **need for larger clinical trials** to establish **long-term safety and efficacy**

No research has been identified in relation to role of antiproliferative agents in the management of OSMF , erythroplakia, PVL and palatal lesions in reverse smokers.

Topical bleomycin shows **promising efficacy** in reducing **oral leukoplakia lesion size and severity** through its **cytotoxic action on dysplastic cells**. While **well-tolerated,** concerns about **systemic toxicity and local side effects** highlight the need for **larger clinical trials** to establish its **long-term safety and optimal dosing**.

Metformin

Metformin, commonly used for diabetes management, has shown promise in inhibiting cancer progression by targeting the mTOR signaling pathway.

Tsao et al. (2021) [140] investigated metformin's role in inhibiting the mTOR signaling pathway to slow the progression of oral premalignant lesions. Despite promising results, the study had several limitations. Firstly, the sample size was small, limiting the generalizability of the findings. Secondly, the study duration may not have been long enough to assess long-term efficacy and safety, especially in preventing malignant transformation. Additionally, variations in dosage, patient metabolism, and underlying health conditions could influence metformin's effectiveness, requiring further investigation. The study also lacked comparative analysis with other chemopreventive agents, making it unclear whether metformin is superior or merely complementary. Lastly, while metformin is cost-effective, potential side effects such as gastrointestinal discomfort and lactic acidosis need further evaluation in high-risk populations. Larger, well-controlled clinical trials are necessary to validate these findings and establish standardized treatment protocols.

No research has been identified in relation to role of metformin in the management of OSMF , erythroplakia, PVL and palatal lesions in reverse smokers.

Metformin shows **potential in slowing oral premalignant lesion progression** by **inhibiting the mTOR pathway**, but its **long-term efficacy and safety remain uncertain** due to **small sample size and study limitations**. Further **large-scale trials** are needed to confirm its **effectiveness, optimal dosage, and comparative benefits** in chemoprevention.

ADJUNCT THERAPIES

PHYSICAL THERAPY

MOUTH OPENING EXERCISES

Physical therapy plays a vital role in managing trismus and improving mouth opening in individuals with Oral Submucous Fibrosis (OSMF). Since OSMF leads to progressive fibrosis and restricted oral movement, targeted exercises and therapeutic interventions can help enhance jaw mobility, alleviate pain, and improve oral function. Various physical therapy techniques, including mouth-opening exercises, ultrasound therapy, and mechanical devices, have been explored for their effectiveness in managing OSMF.

Mouth-Opening Exercises

Mouth-opening exercises are a non-invasive and cost-effective way to maintain and improve oral mobility in OSMF patients. These exercises aim to stretch the fibrotic tissues, enhance jaw movement, and prevent further restriction. Chitlange et al. (2023)[141] emphasized that physiotherapy, including jaw stretching exercises and guided physical therapy, is crucial in managing moderate to severe OSMF. However, while these exercises are widely recommended, their role is often underutilized due to a lack of standardized protocols for physiotherapists. Regular mouth-opening exercises, when combined with other therapeutic modalities, can significantly enhance treatment outcomes.

ULTRASOUND THERAPY

Ultrasound therapy has gained attention as a **non-invasive therapeutic option** for improving mouth opening in OSMF patients. This technique **delivers sound waves deep into the tissues**, promoting **blood circulation, reducing fibrosis, and improving tissue elasticity**. Senthilkumar et al. (2020) [142] conducted a study comparing **jaw-opening exercises alone versus ultrasound therapy combined with exercises**. Their findings revealed that **patients receiving ultrasound therapy showed greater improvements in mouth opening**, highlighting its **potential as an adjunct treatment**. By reducing **inflammation and fibrosis progression**, ultrasound therapy may provide a **long-term benefit** for patients experiencing severe trismus.

MOUTH OPENING SCREWS

Mechanical devices such as **mouth-opening screws** apply **gradual, controlled force** on the **temporomandibular joints (TMJ) and surrounding tissues**, helping to **break fibrotic bands** and **increase inter-incisal distance**. Chandran et al. (2017)[143] demonstrated that **mouth-opening screws significantly improved mouth opening**, particularly when **used in combination with other treatments**. Sharma et al. (2020)[144] further validated these findings, reporting **an increase of 2-4 cm in mouth opening** over **4-6 months**, especially in **early to moderate** OSMF cases. Additionally, Mehta et al. (2021)[145] found that **combining mouth-opening screws with corticosteroid therapy** led to **superior outcomes**, as the mechanical stretching effect complemented the **anti-inflammatory action of corticosteroids**. However, Singh et al. (2023)[146] cautioned that **advanced OSMF cases may experience discomfort or difficulty adjusting to the device**, necessitating **careful patient selection and regular monitoring** to optimize results.

LASERS

Laser-based surgical interventions have shown promise in managing oral leukoplakia (OL) by potentially reducing recurrence rates compared to conventional surgical excision. Bhattarai et al. (2024)[147] identified clinicopathological factors such as female sex, advanced age, nonhomogeneous OL, and inadequate surgical margins as significant predictors of recurrence, emphasizing the need for close post-treatment monitoring. Rui Luo et al. (2024)[148] conducted a network meta-analysis of various laser modalities, identifying Er,Cr:YSGG laser as the most effective in reducing OL recurrence while also minimizing postoperative discomfort. The study highlighted Er:YAG and CO_2 laser combined with photodynamic therapy (PDT) as viable alternatives, particularly for non-homogeneous OLK, although further high-quality randomized controlled trials (RCTs) are needed. However, in the context of proliferative verrucous leukoplakia (PVL), laser therapy has yielded mixed results. Cobb et al. (2024)[149] reported ineffectiveness of CO_2 laser ablation, with lesions recurring and expanding over two decades. In contrast, Bombeccari et al. (2024)[150] observed successful disease control with diode laser excision, particularly in PVL lesions associated with HPV-16 infection, suggesting that patient-specific factors influence treatment success.

For erythroplakia, laser therapy appears to be a minimally invasive and effective option. Condor et al. (2023)[151] reviewed 22 studies and concluded that CO_2 laser treatment offers advantages such as precise tissue removal, minimal bleeding, and faster healing for oral leukoplakia, erythroplakia, and lichen planus. Sattayut et al. (2023)[152] further emphasized the role of laser therapy in reducing dysplastic progression and recurrence, particularly CO_2 laser ablation, diode lasers, and PDT, which have demonstrated effectiveness in lowering the risk of malignant transformation. However, lesion size remains a key predictor of recurrence, reinforcing the need for long-term clinical studies to establish standardized treatment protocols. The potential integration of laser therapy into primary care settings could facilitate early intervention and improved patient outcomes for erythroplakia management.

In oral submucous fibrosis (OSMF), laser therapy is gaining recognition as a non-invasive treatment option for improving mouth opening and oral function. Gondivkar et al. (2020) [153]systematically analyzed seven clinical studies and reported significant improvements in trismus relief (6.84 mm–23.7 mm increase in mouth opening) using laser therapy, along with reduced burning sensation and increased tongue mobility. Aparna et al. (2023)[154] conducted a comparative study between low-level laser therapy (LLLT) and intralesional steroid injections, concluding that LLLT provided better immediate results, while intralesional steroids yielded superior long-term effects. However, both treatment modalities failed to significantly alter fibrotic bands, suggesting that laser therapy should be integrated into a multimodal treatment plan for OSMF. While lasers offer promising short-term benefits, a combination approach with pharmacological and rehabilitative therapies remains essential for sustained functional improvement and prevention of malignant transformation.

CRYOSURGERY

Cryosurgery has emerged as a minimally invasive alternative for managing oral leukoplakia and erythroplakia, offering advantages such as reduced postoperative discomfort and satisfactory lesion resolution. Kumar et al. (2017)[155] reported on the clinical applicability of cryosurgery using refrigerant gas, emphasizing its potential as an effective treatment option. However, long-term follow-up studies are needed to assess its efficacy in preventing recurrence and reducing malignant transformation risks when compared to conventional treatment modalities such as scalpel excision or laser therapy.

Pandey et al. (2023) [156]conducted a comparative evaluation of four surgical modalities—cryosurgery, scalpel and blade surgery, diode laser surgery, and CO_2 laser surgery—for treating oral potentially malignant disorders, including erythroplakia. While all four techniques demonstrated effectiveness, cryotherapy yielded superior clinical outcomes in terms of postoperative pain and edema reduction, making it a promising option for enhancing patient comfort. Given its non-invasive nature and potential for effective lesion control, cryotherapy may serve as a viable alternative to conventional surgical excision, particularly in cases where minimizing post-treatment morbidity is a priority. Further research is needed to standardize treatment protocols and establish long-term recurrence rates.

PHOTODYNAMIC THERAPY

Photodynamic therapy (PDT) has emerged as a minimally invasive and effective treatment for Oral Potentially Malignant Disorders (OPMDs) such as oral leukoplakia (OL), proliferative verrucous leukoplakia (PVL), erythroplakia, and oral submucous fibrosis (OSMF). PDT involves the application of a photosensitizing agent, which, upon exposure to a specific wavelength of light, produces reactive oxygen species (ROS) that selectively destroy abnormal cells while preserving surrounding healthy tissue. This approach is gaining traction due to its targeted action, reduced morbidity, and potential to prevent malignant transformation.

Oral leukoplakia (OL) is the most common precancerous lesion, with a significant risk of malignant transformation (MT), especially in non-homogeneous OL and cases with inadequate surgical margins (Bhattarai et al., 2024)[147]. Traditional treatments, including surgical excision and laser ablation, show varying recurrence rates. Rui Luo et al. (2024)[148] conducted a network meta-analysis comparing different surgical and laser approaches for OL management. The study found that CO_2 laser combined with PDT showed promising results in reducing recurrence rates compared to surgical excision alone. This suggests that PDT may play a crucial role in enhancing treatment efficacy and reducing lesion recurrence.

For proliferative verrucous leukoplakia (PVL), a high-risk OPMD with persistent and multifocal lesions, standard treatments often fail to provide long-term control. Cobb et al. (2024)[149] reported a case of PVL managed with CO_2 laser, but the lesion persisted and expanded despite multiple interventions. Bombeccari et al. (2024)[150] detailed a case where diode laser excision resulted in favorable outcomes for a PVL patient with HPV-16-associated mild dysplasia. These findings indicate that while lasers provide effective lesion removal, PDT may serve as an adjunct therapy to prevent recurrence and target field cancerization effects in PVL.

PDT in Erythroplakia

Erythroplakia, due to its high malignant transformation rate, demands aggressive intervention. Condor et al. (2023) reviewed CO_2 laser therapy's efficacy in treating potentially malignant oral lesions, including erythroplakia. While CO_2 laser therapy demonstrated effective lesion ablation with minimal postoperative discomfort, the integration of PDT with laser treatment could further enhance dysplastic cell eradication while reducing recurrence rates. Sattayut et al. (2023) [152]emphasized that CO_2 laser, diode laser, and PDT are all promising strategies for erythroplakia management, but lesion size remains a key predictor of recurrence. Future research should explore combining laser and PDT approaches to optimize patient outcomes.

PDT in Oral Submucous Fibrosis (OSMF)

In OSMF, a chronic, progressive disorder leading to fibrosis and restricted mouth opening, PDT may offer a novel therapeutic strategy. While physical therapy, ultrasound, and mouth-opening screws have been explored for improving oral function (Chitlange et al., 2023;[141] Senthilkumar et al., 2020), [142]low-level laser therapy (LLLT) and PDT could potentially modulate fibrosis and enhance treatment outcomes. Gondivkar et al. (2020)[153] reported that laser therapy (LT) significantly improved mouth opening in OSMF patients, suggesting that PDT may provide additional anti-fibrotic effects when combined with other interventions.

SURGICAL MANAGEMENT

Surgical management of oral cavity premalignancy requires a comprehensive, risk-stratified approach to optimize patient outcomes. Wei Liu et al. (2023)[158] emphasize the importance of identifying high-risk lesions to prevent malignant transformation and highlight the need for well-designed randomized controlled trials (RCTs) to establish evidence-based surgical guidelines. Future research should focus on standardizing risk assessment models and comparing surgical techniques to refine strategies and improve prognosis

The surgical management of proliferative verrucous leukoplakia (PVL), as discussed by Abadie et al. (2015)[159], includes scalpel excision, laser ablation, electrocautery, cryoablation, and photodynamic therapy, with scalpel excision being the preferred method due to its ability to provide histological evaluation. Given the multifocal and recurrent nature of PVL, patients often undergo multiple treatment modalities throughout the disease course. Similarly, surgical excision is the gold standard for erythroplakia management, as noted by Awadallah et al. (2014)[160], due to its high malignant transformation rate (MTR). The authors recommend excision to the submucosal level in non-tongue lesions and to the superficial muscular level for tongue involvement, emphasizing early surgical intervention, risk factor modification, and long-term surveillance.

For Oral Submucous Fibrosis (OSMF), Gavali et al. (2022)[161] highlight various surgical approaches, including fibrotic band excision, coronoidectomy, and reconstructive procedures using grafts or flaps. These interventions aim to restore mouth opening and improve patient quality of life, but they must be accompanied by cessation of etiological factors such as areca nut chewing to prevent recurrence. The review underscores the need for adjunctive medical therapies and a multidisciplinary approach to optimize long-term outcomes. While surgery remains a key component of premalignancy management, ongoing research is crucial to establish optimal treatment protocols, minimize recurrence, and reduce the risk of malignant transformation across different oral potentially malignant disorders (OPMDs)

Protocol for Management of Tobacco Associated OPMDS

LEUKOLAKIA

The primary aim in the management of oral leukoplakia is to monitor and prevent the onset of oral cancer. Various treatment protocols have been proposed, including medical management (topical or systemic therapies), clinical observation (strict surveillance with periodic biopsies), and surgical intervention. However, there is no universal consensus on the most appropriate approach, as none of the studied medical treatments (vitamin A, beta-carotene, bleomycin) have been definitively proven to prevent malignant transformation. Additionally, chemo-preventive agents have demonstrated significant toxicity, limiting their widespread use. While pharmacological management may help in reducing or resolving leukoplakia in the short term, recurrence rates remain high, necessitating long-term monitoring.

Patient assessment begins with a thorough history, including lesion duration, tobacco or alcohol use, systemic diseases, and previous oral lesions or malignancies. Clinical examination evaluates the lesion's location, size, texture, and any ulceration, nodularity, or induration, along with cervical lymph node assessment. Diagnostic workup includes exfoliative cytology for preliminary screening, followed by biopsy and histopathological evaluation to determine dysplasia severity. Adjunctive diagnostic tools such as toluidine blue staining and autofluorescence help identify high-risk lesions that may require more aggressive intervention. Pharmacological management plays a crucial role, particularly for early-stage or non-surgical lesions. Antioxidants such as beta-carotene, lycopene, and vitamin A help reduce oxidative stress and potentially inhibit dysplasia progression. Retinoids, including isotretinoin and fenretinide, modulate epithelial differentiation and reduce keratinocyte proliferation, showing efficacy in reversing dysplastic changes. Topical bleomycin has been explored for its cytotoxic effects on dysplastic cells, effectively reducing lesion size, though concerns about systemic toxicity remain. Immunomodulatory agents such as imiquimod, a toll-like receptor agonist, have demonstrated potential in stimulating an anti-tumor immune response and improving lesion resolution. Additionally, metformin, an mTOR pathway inhibitor, has been investigated for its ability to slow oral leukoplakia lesion progression, though further research is needed to validate its efficacy. Systemic agents like sirolimus and levamisole have also been studied for their immunomodulatory effects, with some symptomatic improvements observed. However, their long-term safety and effectiveness remain under investigation.

Despite these pharmacological options, surgical intervention remains the primary treatment for high-risk leukoplakia, especially in cases with moderate to severe dysplasia. Techniques such as scalpel excision, CO2 laser ablation, cryotherapy, and photodynamic therapy are commonly employed. While surgical removal may reduce malignant transformation risk, some cases may not be suitable for excision, necessitating laser ablation or strict observation. Laser therapy offers advantages in areas where surgery is not feasible, such as anatomically challenging locations or in patients with contraindications for surgical procedures. It is also associated with reduced postoperative discomfort and quicker healing times. Regular follow-up is essential, with low-risk lesions monitored every 3–6 months and high-risk lesions requiring closer surveillance with periodic re-biopsies. Long-term patient care includes lifestyle modifications such as smoking and alcohol cessation, nutritional counseling, and education on early signs of malignant transformation. Psychological support may also be necessary to address patient concerns and improve compliance with management protocols.

Treatment Modalities

Non-Invasive Chemoprevention

- **Antioxidants:**
  - **Spirulina (1 g/day, 6 months)**: Most effective among natural compounds..
  - **Lycopene (8 mg/day, 3 months)**: Significant improvement with minimal toxicity.
  - **Curcumin (1% topical gel, twice daily, 12 weeks)**: Marked lesion reduction.
  - **Beta-carotene + Vitamin C (30 mg + 500 mg/day, 6 months)**: Modest effects, lower complete response rates.
  - **Comprehensive Vitamin Therapy (A, C, and E, 3–6 months)**: Limited efficacy.
  - **Retinoids (0.5–1 mg/kg/day, 3 months or 0.1% gel, twice daily, 12 weeks)**: Effective but high recurrence and adverse effects.

Targeted Pharmacological Therapies

- **mTOR Inhibitors:**
  - **Metformin (500–1000 mg/day, 12 months)**: Effective mTOR inhibitor reducing lesion progression.
- **EGFR and COX-2 Inhibitors:**
  - **Erlotinib (150 mg/day) + Celecoxib (400 mg/day, 6 months)**: 63% histologic response, but limited follow-up data.
- **Cytotoxic Agents:**
  - **Bleomycin (Topical, 2016, Shetty et al.)**: Effective but high toxicity (mucosal ulceration, fibrosis).
- **Immunomodulatory Drugs:**
  - **Imiquimod (Topical, TLR agonist)**: Enhances immune response but requires further studies.
  - **Sirolimus & Levamisole**: Immunomodulatory effects under investigation.

Management Strategy

If a patient presents with oral leukoplakia, management will be determined based on risk level:

- **Step 1: Initial Assessment**
  - Conduct a thorough history and physical examination.
  - Identify risk factors (tobacco, alcohol, HPV, betel quid use).
- Toluidine blue staining or autofluorescence, followed by biopsy for histopathological assessment, helps evaluate leukoplakia. Biopsy samples are typically stained with Hematoxylin and Eosin to determine dysplasia severity and detect malignant changes. Immunohistochemistry may be used to identify cancer-associated molecular markers.
- **Step 2: Risk Stratification & First-Line Management**
  - **Low-Risk (No/Mild Dysplasia):**
    - **Preferred:** Antioxidants such as Lycopene (8 mg/day, 3 months) or Curcumin (1% gel, twice daily, 12 weeks).
    - **Alternative:** Comprehensive vitamin therapy (Vitamin A, C, E).
    - **Follow-up:** Every 3–6 months.
  - **Moderate to High-Risk (Moderate/Severe Dysplasia):**
    - **Preferred:** Targeted therapy with Metformin (500–1000 mg/day, 12 months) or Laser Excision.
    - **Alternative:** Retinoids (oral or topical) for epithelial modulation.
    - **Follow-up:** Close monitoring every 3 months with periodic biopsies.

  Usually mild to moderate leukoplakia often corresponds to homogeneous leukoplakia, severe dysplasia is more frequent in non-homogeneous types.

  - **Recurrent or Extensive:**
    - **Preferred:** Laser surgery combined with chemoprevention (Curcumin, Lycopene, or Metformin).
    - **Alternative:** Targeted pharmacological therapy (Erlotinib + Celecoxib).
    - **Follow-up:** Intensive surveillance every 1–3 months.
- **Step 3: Surgical Intervention for High-Risk Cases**
  - **Laser-Based Surgery (Preferred):**
    - **Er,Cr:YSGG and Er:YAG lasers**: Reduced recurrence, minimized bleeding and pain.
    - **Photodynamic Therapy (PDT)**: Well-tolerated, effective lesion reduction.
    - **Cryosurgery**: Less invasive, fewer complications.

    - **Conventional Excision (Gold Standard for Severe Dysplasia).**
- **Step 4: Long-Term Surveillance & Prevention**
    - **Lifestyle Modifications:** Smoking and alcohol cessation, nutritional counseling.
    - **Regular Monitoring:**
        - **Low-Risk:** Follow-up every 3–6 months.
        - **High-Risk:** Follow-up every 1–3 months with periodic re-biopsies.
    - **Psychosocial Support:** Counseling for compliance and risk reduction.

This protocol integrates pharmacological interventions with surgical and preventive strategies to optimize patient outcomes, reduce malignant transformation risks, and provide a comprehensive approach to the management of oral leukoplakia.

PVL

The management and treatment of PVL is particularly challenging in the last decade, different approaches have been proposed to reduce the high incidence of oral cancer among patients affected by PVL. To date, none of the treatments, (surgery, laser ablation, retinoids, photodynamic therapy and chemo¬therapy) have proven to be effective in reducing oral cancer development in these patients . Despite the lack of evidence on efficacy, surgical treatment is the most frequent intervention adopted in the management of PVL When PVL is characterised by small lesions, and if the area is discrete, excision may be attempted, but the patient should be aware that ongoing follow-up will be necessary due to high oral cancer risk and risk of lesion recurrence (71%) Most PVL cases demonstrate large lesions and involve multifocal non contiguous areas. A recent systematic review reported the overall recurrence rate of PVL to all treatment modalities is approximately 85% without any reduction in cancer incidence For all these reasons, surgical excision in extensive PVL may be considered an impractical and unnecessary aggressive treatment option

Multimodal Treatment Approach:

- Due to PVL's aggressive and recurrent nature, a single treatment modality is often insufficient. A combination of surgical excision and adjuvant therapies may yield the most favorable outcomes.

Surgical Intervention:

- Surgical excision (scalpel-based) is preferred when lesions are small and localized, primarily due to its ability to provide histopathological confirmation.
- For larger, multifocal, or non-contiguous lesions, surgery may be impractical. In such cases, less invasive approaches like laser ablation may be considered.
- Diode lasers may offer a conservative alternative, while CO_2 lasers have shown limited long-term efficacy.

Adjuvant and Alternative Therapies:

- Retinoids: These may promote cellular differentiation but are not curative, especially in high-grade dysplasia cases.
- Photodynamic Therapy (PDT): Although promising for oral verrucous hyperplasia and erythroleukoplakia, its role in PVL remains uncertain and requires further study.
- Immunomodulatory Therapy (e.g., Imiquimod): Case reports suggest potential efficacy, but the lack of large-scale studies limits its routine application.

Long-Term Monitoring and Patient Education:

- Regular follow-up is crucial due to PVL's high recurrence rate (up to 85%) and malignant transformation risk.
- Patients should be counseled on the importance of routine surveillance, smoking cessation, alcohol reduction, and awareness of early malignant changes.

Tailored Treatment Plans:

- Due to the variability in lesion size, location, and patient-specific factors, management should be personalized. A multidisciplinary approach involving surgeons, oncologists, and oral medicine specialists is recommended.

ERYTHROPLAKIA

Owing to the highest risk of malignant transformation early treatment is crucial. Surgical excision is the treatment of choice. There is lack of studies on follow-up following surgical excision and treatment outcomes. There are no guidelines on the exact margin to excise, this is often dictated by the degree of cellular atypia identified. Carbon dioxide laser excision has been used recently, as an alternative to scalpel excision. This has been associated with more favourable healing of the area and post-operative comfort. The rate of recurrence following excision is unknown, however, the size of the excised lesion has been shown to be a significant predictive factor [77]Other therapies including vitamin A, retinoids, bleomycin and mixed tea have not yielded favourable results to advocate their use. Cessation of recreational habits associated with higher risk of malignant transformation should be recommended There is no suggested follow-up interval for erythroplakia. An increase in size, high risk recreational habits (smoking/alcohol), high risk sites (ventral tongue and floor of mouth), change in clinical appearance and the development of symptoms may dictate re-biopsy of a lesion. A clinical photograph taken at subsequent appointments is useful to objectively assess for any changes in appearance of the lesion [77]

Management Strategy

Diagnosis and Initial Assessment:

- Patient History: Start by taking a comprehensive medical, social, and dental history, focusing on risk factors such as tobacco use, alcohol consumption, and a history of previous oral lesions.
- Clinical Examination: Perform a thorough oral examination to assess the size, location, and characteristics of the erythroplakia lesion. Erythroplakia typically appears as a red, velvety patch on the oral mucosa, often without a raised or indurated border.
- Imaging and Documentation: Take high-resolution clinical photographs for baseline documentation and comparison during follow-up visits.

Biopsy and Histopathological Examination:

- Indication: A biopsy is essential to establish a definitive diagnosis since erythroplakia has a high risk of malignant transformation.
- Biopsy Technique: Use an incisional or excisional biopsy, depending on lesion size and location. The sample should include both the lesion and adjacent normal tissue to assess the degree of dysplasia or presence of carcinoma.
- Histopathological Analysis: The biopsy specimen should be evaluated for the presence of dysplasia, carcinoma in situ, or invasive squamous cell carcinoma (SCC). Approximately 90% of erythroplakia cases show some degree of dysplasia or SCC.

Treatment Plan:

- **Based on Histopathological Findings:**
    - No Dysplasia or Mild Dysplasia: Consider careful monitoring with regular follow-ups (every 3–6 months) and patient education on risk factor modification (smoking and alcohol cessation).

- Moderate to Severe Dysplasia or SCC: Proceed with surgical excision as the primary treatment.

Surgical Management:

- Scalpel Excision:
    - Considered the gold standard due to its ability to completely remove the lesion and provide tissue for histopathological evaluation.
    - Margins should be dictated by the degree of cellular atypia, often extending to the submucosal or superficial muscular level (especially on the tongue).
- **Laser Excision (CO_2 or Diode Laser):**
    - Useful when the lesion is in a location that makes scalpel excision challenging or when minimizing bleeding is crucial.
    - Advantages: Reduced intraoperative bleeding, faster healing, and less postoperative discomfort.
    - Limitations: Limited ability to evaluate margins histologically.

Adjuvant and Alternative Therapies:

- Photodynamic Therapy (PDT):
    - Considered for patients who are not suitable candidates for surgery.
    - Uses 5-ALA as a photosensitizer followed by light activation.
    - Effective in cases with mild to moderate dysplasia but lacks long-term outcome data.
- Medical Management:
    - Not typically recommended due to limited efficacy. Options like retinoids and topical agents (e.g., imiquimod) may be considered in select cases but are generally adjuncts rather than primary treatments.

Postoperative Care and Follow-Up:

- Follow-Up Schedule: Initially every 3 months for the first year, then every 6 months thereafter.
- Monitoring for Recurrence: High recurrence rates (around 30% reported), so vigilance is necessary.
- Lifestyle Modifications: Smoking and alcohol cessation are critical to reduce recurrence and transformation risk.
- Patient Education: Inform about the signs of recurrence or malignant transformation (e.g., ulceration, increased size, pain).

Long-Term Management:

- Recurrence Management: If recurrence occurs, reassess the lesion with a biopsy and consider re-excision or alternative therapies like laser ablation.
- Multidisciplinary Approach: Collaboration with oral surgeons, pathologists, and oncologists is essential for managing cases with confirmed malignancy.

OSMF

Patients should be counselled on the continued use of Areca nut chewing and its role in the aetiopathogenesis and risk of malignant transformation and should be encouraged to stop the habit. OSMF carries a significant global disease burden and primary prevention is a key focus of government strategy in countries within the Indian subcontinent. Approaches such as banning Areca plant products and their preparations, as well as education on the harmful effects of Areca nut chewing have been demonstrated to be useful in primary prevention at both individual and population levels . OSMF often presents late creating a management dilemma. Conservative management: In the moderate to severe stages of OSMF, the degree of fibrosis is irreversible, and treatment is primarily symptomatic. Conservative management for progressive reduction of mouth opening involves physical therapy. Various exercises aimed at stretching the tissues and strengthening the muscles of mastication are advised. Custom made devices may also be useful in reducing trismus. Patients are encouraged to massage the muscles of mastication. Oral hygiene should be reinforced as patients with OSMF display higher levels of dental diseases such as periodontal disease, dental caries and halitosis Patients complaining of general oral discomfort can be prescribed anesthetic. In more advanced stages of OSMF, intralesional corticosteroid injections have been useful in reducing trismus but with limited success . Other topical treatments such as hyaluronidase may be useful and have a synergistic effect when used in combination with other topical treatments. Hyaluronidase catalyses the degradation of hyaluronic acid, a component of collagen. Other fibrinolytic therapies include the use of chemotrypsin and collagenase. Interferon gamma is a recognised antifibrotic cytokine and intralesional injection has demonstrated therapeutic effect. Intralesional application of placental extracts has also been demonstrated to be efficacious Other therapies aim to promote oral mucosal blood f low. Pentoxyphyline is a drug that alters fibroblast physiology and also improves tissue oxygenation by improving peripheral blood flow. It has been shown to provide symptomatic relief to patients with OSMF. Agents such Beta-adrenergic agonist drugs have a vasodilatory effect and also have been demonstrated to provide symptomatic relief Oral Potentially Malignant Disorders: Healthcare Professional Training 10. Oral Submucous Fibrosis The use of antioxidants, nutrients, micronutrients therapy (AONMT) are aimed at improving the nutritional status of patients with OSMF and are used in combination with vitamin and mineral supplementation. Agents such as Beta-carotene and lycopene are used to promote cellular health and have a protective effect with regards to the carcinogenic process . There exists no globally accepted conservative management technique/s for OSMF. Kerr et al. found a low grade of evidence to support recommendations for the management of OSF.. Surgical Management: Surgical treatment may be indicated in severe cases of trismus and aims to improve mouth opening and masticatory and oral health . The surgical approach usually involves removal of the fibrosed tissue and after care is aimed at maintaining opening after removal and muscle release . Simple excision of the fibrosed bands exacerbates the condition, as iatrogenic trauma from the surgical process leads to subsequent fibrosis Chronic trismus as a result of OSMF can lead to physiological changes in the temporalis tendon and skin grafting procedures may help to resolve this, for example a Split-thickness skin grafting following bilateral temporalis myotomy or a coronoidectomy . These are extensive surgical procedures and should not be undertaken lightly, but may alleviate the symptoms of trismus . Myotomy of other masticatory muscles may also be considered Various flaps such as the nasolabial flap and its modifications (the extended nasolabial flap/ winged nasolabial flap/ facial artery-based nasolabial flap) are used to resurface intraoral defects after the above procedures . These procedures result in aesthetically compromising facial scarring, however, in the Indian subcontinent it is widely applied due the simplicity of the procedure and the high success rate Free flaps are extensive surgical procedures primarily used in the management of oral squamous cell carcinoma . The radial forearm free flap involves harvesting tissue from the forearm and is considered to be the gold standard surgical approach in the management of severe recalcitrant OSMF . To avoid recurrence following surgery, postoperative physiotherapy is essential to maintain mouth opening. Physical therapy methods post-operatively are similar to those involved in the conservative management of OSMF Preoperative planning involves clinical, radiological and histopathological screening

Management Stratergies

Diagnosis and Initial Assessment:

- Patient History:
  - Document the patient's habit history, focusing on areca nut chewing, tobacco use, alcohol consumption, and any symptoms such as burning sensation, difficulty opening the mouth (trismus), or altered speech.
  - Explore any previous treatments or interventions for oral lesions.
- Clinical Examination:
  - Assess the oral cavity for fibrotic bands, blanching of the mucosa, reduced mouth opening, and palpable fibrotic tissue.
  - Measure the inter-incisal distance to evaluate the degree of trismus.
- Risk Factor Counseling:
  - Educate the patient about the role of areca nut chewing and tobacco in the aetiopathogenesis of OSMF and the potential for malignant transformation.
  - Emphasize cessation of areca nut and tobacco use, as continued use increases the risk of malignant transformation.

---

2. Diagnostic Investigations:

- Biopsy:
  - Perform an incisional biopsy for histopathological confirmation, especially in cases where malignancy is suspected.
- Imaging:
  - Consider imaging (like MRI or ultrasound) to assess the extent of fibrosis, particularly in advanced cases.
- Blood Tests:
  - Evaluate nutritional deficiencies, as many OSMF patients present with micronutrient deficiencies.

---

3. **Conservative Management**:

- Physical Therapy:
  - Encourage mouth-opening exercises to stretch fibrotic bands and maintain mobility.
  - Use mouth-opening devices such as mouth-opening screws to gradually increase the inter-incisal distance.

- Ultrasound therapy may be used to improve tissue elasticity.

- Nutritional Support:
  - Prescribe antioxidant supplements (e.g., lycopene, beta-carotene, and vitamins A, C, and E) to reduce oxidative stress.
  - Improve the patient's nutritional status with a balanced diet rich in vitamins and minerals.
- Pharmacological Interventions:
  - Corticosteroids:
    - Intralesional injections of corticosteroids (e.g., triamcinolone, dexamethasone) combined with hyaluronidase to reduce fibrosis and inflammation.
    - Topical corticosteroid gels for symptomatic relief of burning sensation.
  - Hyaluronidase:
    - Often combined with corticosteroids to enhance the breakdown of fibrotic tissue.
  - Pentoxifylline:
    - Oral administration (400 mg two to three times daily) to improve blood circulation and reduce fibrosis.
  - Interferon-Gamma:
    - Intralesional injections to reduce fibrotic tissue.
  - Beta-Carotene and Lycopene:
    - Supplements that support cellular health and reduce carcinogenic progression.
  - Other Agents:
    - Use of fibrinolytics (e.g., chymotrypsin, collagenase) for enzymatic degradation of fibrotic bands.
    - Placental extract injections to enhance tissue regeneration.

---

4. Surgical Management (for Severe Cases):

- Indications:
  - Severe trismus (inter-incisal distance <20 mm) not responding to conservative management.
- Procedures:

- Fibrotic Band Excision:
    - Surgical removal of fibrotic bands followed by reconstruction using flaps (e.g., nasolabial flap or radial forearm free flap).
- Coronoidectomy:
    - Performed when temporalis muscle involvement is significant.
- Myotomy:
    - Release of masticatory muscle tension to improve mouth opening.
- Laser Ablation:
    - CO_2 or diode laser to excise fibrotic tissue with reduced bleeding.
- Cryotherapy:
    - Controlled freezing to reduce fibrotic tissue.

5. Postoperative and Long-Term Care:

- Postoperative Physiotherapy:
    - Vital to maintain mouth opening following surgery to prevent recurrence.
    - Include structured physiotherapy with mouth-opening exercises and use of customized devices.
- Monitoring:
    - Regular follow-up every 3 months for the first year, then biannually to monitor for recurrence or malignant transformation.
- Patient Education:
    - Emphasize the importance of maintaining oral hygiene as OSMF patients are prone to dental issues like caries and periodontal disease.
    - Educate on early signs of malignancy, such as non-healing ulcers or changes in the lesion.

---

6. Prognosis and Follow-Up:

- OSMF is a chronic, progressive disease with a potential risk of malignant transformation (about 7-13%).
- Long-term follow-up is crucial, focusing on lifestyle modifications, nutritional support, and monitoring for malignant changes.
- Encourage patients to adhere to oral hygiene practices and physical therapy exercises to maintain improved mouth opening.

Palatal Lesions in Reverse Smokers

Management is dependent on the histological diagnosis. Lesions with moderate to severe dysplasia may undergo surgical excision. The exact malignant transformation rate of PLRS is unknown due to the lack of studies. Similarly, the recurrence rates after treatment are also unknown. Van Der Eb et al. , concluded that reverse chutta smoking was one of the major determinants for palatal cancer A dose frequency relationship is assumed, however cannot be confirmed due to the paucity of studies.

Management Stratergies

Initial Assessment:

- Medical and Habit History: Document smoking practices (reverse smoking), frequency, duration, and other risk factors like alcohol use.
- Clinical Examination:
    - Check for color changes (keratosis, erythema), ulceration, nodularity, induration, and symmetry.
- Risk Assessment: Evaluate additional risk factors and family history of oral cancer.

Diagnostic Workup:

- Biopsy: Mandatory for histopathological confirmation, particularly if the lesion shows signs of dysplasia or malignancy.
- Imaging: Use MRI or CT if there's suspicion of bone involvement.
- Cytology: As an adjunct to biopsy, use brush biopsy or exfoliative cytology for early screening.

Patient Counseling and Education:

- Smoking Cessation: Educate patients on the risks of reverse smoking and encourage quitting.
- Reassurance: Explain that benign smoker's palate often resolves spontaneously with smoking cessation.
- Oral Hygiene: Emphasize the importance of maintaining good oral hygiene to reduce secondary infections.

Combined Treatment Approach:

Conservative and Pharmacological Management:

- Observation: For benign lesions, monitor for spontaneous resolution post-smoking cessation.
- Topical Therapy:
  - Curcumin Oral Gel: Apply via a custom-made acrylic palatal plate, which has shown to reduce lesion size.
  - Antioxidant Gels: Lycopene and vitamin-enriched formulations may enhance mucosal health.
- Anti-Inflammatory Treatment:
  - Topical Steroids: Use for significant inflammation or discomfort.
- Adjunctive Supplements:
  - Antioxidants (Vitamin A, C, E): To improve mucosal health and reduce oxidative stress.

Surgical Intervention (if indicated):

- Indications: Persistent lesions, moderate to severe dysplasia, or carcinoma in situ.
- Options:
  - Excision: Complete removal of dysplastic areas.
  - Laser Ablation: Suitable for small, localized lesions.
- Postoperative Care: Smoking cessation reinforcement, oral hygiene instructions, and regular follow-up.

Long-Term Follow-Up:

- Regular clinical exams every 3-6 months.
- Repeat biopsy if lesions persist despite cessation or exhibit suspicious changes.
- Multidisciplinary collaboration with oral surgeons and oncologists for complex cases.

ROLE OF ORAL PHYSICIANS IN MEDICAL MANAGEMENT

Oral Potentially Malignant Disorders (OPMDs) require early detection, a multidisciplinary approach, and patient education to prevent malignant transformation and optimize patient outcomes. Dentists and physicians play a critical role in identifying, diagnosing, and managing OPMDs through collaborative strategies.

Early Detection and Intervention

Early detection of OPMDs such as oral leukoplakia (OL), erythroplakia, proliferative verrucous leukoplakia (PVL), and oral submucous fibrosis (OSMF) significantly impacts treatment success and prognosis. Since OL and PVL have a high risk of malignant transformation, timely identification and histopathological examination are crucial (Bhattarai et al., 2024). Dentists are often the first to detect suspicious oral lesions during routine examinations, emphasizing the importance of oral cancer screenings in dental practice (Rui Luo et al., 2024). Physicians, particularly otolaryngologists and oral medicine specialists, play a complementary role in confirming diagnoses and determining systemic risk factors such as HPV infection, tobacco use, and betel nut chewing (Bombeccari et al., 2024).

Effective intervention strategies include:

- Photodynamic Therapy (PDT): Studies show that PDT combined with CO_2 laser therapy is effective in reducing recurrence rates in OL and PVL (Condor et al., 2023; Sattayut et al., 2023).
- Cryotherapy: Cryosurgery offers a minimally invasive alternative, reducing postoperative discomfort and ensuring lesion resolution, but requires further long-term studies (Kumar et al., 2017; Pandey et al., 2023).
- Low-Level Laser Therapy (LLLT) for OSMF: LLLT and ultrasound therapy are promising modalities for improving mouth opening and reducing fibrosis in OSMF patients (Gondivkar et al., 2020; Senthilkumar et al., 2020)

Multidisciplinary Approach in Managing OPMDs

A multidisciplinary approach involving dentists, physicians, oncologists, physiotherapists, and nutritionists ensures comprehensive OPMD management. Each specialist contributes uniquely:Dentists: Perform oral screenings, biopsies, laser therapy, and prosthetic rehabilitation post-treatment Oral Medicine Specialists: Confirm diagnosis, perform advanced imaging, and guide non-surgical interventions. Oncologists: Monitor high-risk lesions and provide radiotherapy or chemotherapy in cases of malignant transformation. Physiotherapists: Assist in jaw mobility rehabilitation for OSMF patients through mouth-opening exercises, ultrasound therapy, and mouth-opening screws (Chitlange et al., 2023; Chandran et al., 2017). Nutritionists: Provide dietary counseling, especially for OSMF patients, to improve overall nutritional intake and oral health.

Combining these efforts improves patient prognosis and reduces recurrence rates, particularly in cases of erythroplakia and PVL that require frequent monitoring and repeat biopsies (Cobb et al., 2024).

Patient Education and Follow-Up Strategies

Education plays a pivotal role in OPMD management, particularly in regions where betel nut chewing, tobacco use, and HPV-related lesions are prevalent (Sharma et al., 2020; Mehta et al., 2021). Dentists and physicians must:

- Educate patients on risk factors, lifestyle modifications, and early symptoms.
- Implement structured follow-ups, especially for high-risk cases like PVL and erythroplakia, which require long-term surveillance (Singh et al., 2023).
- Utilize digital tracking for recall appointments, lesion monitoring, and biopsy scheduling.
- Encourage compliance with prescribed therapies, including PDT, laser therapy, and cryosurgery.

Follow-up regimens should be customized based on recurrence risk, ensuring that patients with high-risk lesions receive closer monitoring and intervention adjustments.

The **role of dentists and physicians in OPMD management** is **indispensable**, requiring **early detection, multidisciplinary coordination, and patient education**. Advances in **laser therapy, PDT, and physical therapy** have enhanced treatment outcomes, but **regular follow-ups and long-term studies** are crucial to refining management strategies. By **collaborating across specialties and emphasizing patient awareness**, healthcare professionals can significantly **reduce malignant transformation rates and improve quality of life for OPMD patients**.

FUTURE SCOPE

Advanced Diagnostic Techniques: The development of non-invasive and highly sensitive diagnostic tools such as molecular markers, liquid biopsy, and AI-driven imaging can improve early detection and risk assessment of OPMDs.

Targeted Therapies: Future studies should explore precision medicine approaches, focusing on genetic and epigenetic modifications to design patient-specific treatments that minimize recurrence and malignant transformation.

Regenerative Medicine: The role of stem cell therapy and bioengineered tissue grafts in reversing fibrotic changes in OSMF should be further investigated to provide long-term functional restoration.

Personalized Medicine: Advancements in pharmacogenomics can help in identifying patients who will benefit most from specific drug therapies, reducing the trial-and-error approach currently in practice.

Telemedicine and Digital Health: Implementing AI-based teleconsultation services for monitoring OPMD patients in remote areas can improve accessibility and ensure early intervention in high-risk cases.

Preventive Strategies: Stronger public health policies, including mass awareness campaigns, taxation on areca nut and tobacco products, and school-based education programs, can help in primary prevention of OPMDs.

Long-Term Follow-Up Protocols: Establishing standardized follow-up guidelines, including frequency of surveillance and specific criteria for intervention, can help in reducing malignant transformation risks.

CONCLUSION

The medical management of tobacco-associated oral potentially malignant disorders (OPMDs), including conditions such as oral leukoplakia, erythroplakia, proliferative verrucous leukoplakia (PVL), and oral submucous fibrosis (OSMF), remains a critical area of concern in oral healthcare. Despite extensive research and various treatment modalities, there is no single universally accepted approach for managing these conditions. Instead, a multidisciplinary strategy is essential to reduce malignant transformation risk and improve patient outcomes.

The primary focus of management should be on early detection and intervention, as these conditions often present asymptomatically in their initial stages. Tobacco cessation remains the cornerstone of preventive strategies. Given the strong correlation between tobacco use and the development of OPMDs, patients should be counseled on cessation programs, and public health policies should emphasize awareness and education about the harmful effects of tobacco and areca nut consumption. Governments in high-prevalence regions, particularly in the Indian subcontinent, should implement stricter regulations on areca nut products to curb the disease burden.

Medical management of these disorders includes topical and systemic therapies aimed at reducing symptoms and preventing malignant transformation. Various pharmacological agents, including retinoids, vitamin A, beta-carotene, bleomycin, and antifibrotic agents such as hyaluronidase and pentoxifylline, have been investigated for their potential efficacy. However, these treatments have shown mixed results, and none have been proven to significantly prevent cancer onset. Additionally, adverse effects and high recurrence rates post-treatment limit their widespread acceptance in clinical practice.

Given the unpredictable nature of malignant transformation in OPMDs, long-term follow-up and surveillance are crucial. A "wait and see" approach, involving regular clinical and histopathological assessments, is often employed for low-grade lesions. Patients should be monitored at frequent intervals, and any progression in lesion size, texture, or symptoms should prompt re-biopsy and possible intervention.

Clinical photography and digital documentation are valuable tools in tracking disease progression over time. Additionally, genetic and molecular studies may offer future avenues for risk stratification, allowing for more personalized management approaches.

Challenges and Future Directions

Despite advances in treatment modalities, several challenges persist in the management of tobacco-associated OPMDs. The lack of high-quality randomized controlled trials (RCTs) assessing different interventions limits the ability to establish evidence-based guidelines. Furthermore, discrepancies in diagnostic criteria, variations in treatment protocols, and inconsistent follow-up strategies contribute to the heterogeneity in reported outcomes.

Future research should focus on developing targeted therapies based on molecular and genetic markers to predict malignant transformation risk more accurately. Innovations in regenerative medicine, including tissue engineering and stem cell therapy, hold promise for reversing fibrotic changes in conditions like OSMF.

Tobacco-associated OPMDs pose a significant risk for oral cancer development, necessitating proactive management strategies. While surgical intervention remains the primary modality for high-risk lesions, adjunct medical therapies and lifestyle modifications play a vital role in comprehensive patient care. Prevention through tobacco cessation, early diagnosis, and regular follow-up are key to reducing disease progression and improving patient outcomes. Moving forward, a collaborative effort among researchers, clinicians, and public health policymakers is essential to develop standardized guidelines and effective treatment protocols to combat these potentially malignant disorders.

REFERENCES

1. Warnakulasuriya S, Kujan O, Aguirre-Urizar JM, Bagan JV, González Moles MÁ, Kerr AR, et al. Oral potentially malignant disorders: A consensus report from an international seminar on nomenclature and classification, convened by the WHO Collaborating Centre for Oral Cancer. Oral Dis. 2021;27(8):1862-80.
2. Sarode SC, Sarode GS, Tupkari JV. Oral potentially malignant disorders: Precising the definition. *Oral Oncol.* 2012;48(9):759-760.
3. Khan Z, Khan S, Christianson L, Rehman S, Ekwunife O, Samkange-Zeeb F. Smokeless tobacco and oral potentially malignant disorders in South Asia: A systematic review and meta-analysis. *Nicotine Tob Res.* 2018;20(1):12-21.
4. Mortazavi H, Baharvand M, Mehdipour M. Oral potentially malignant disorders: An overview of more than 20 entities. *J Dent Res Dent Clin Dent Prospects.* 2014;8(1):6-14.
5. Arduino PG, Bagan J, El-Naggar AK, Carrozzo M. Urban legends series: Oral leukoplakia. *Oral Dis.* 2013;19(7):642-659.
6. Acharya S, Singh S, Bhatia SK. Association between smokeless tobacco and risk of malignant and premalignant conditions of the oral cavity: A systematic review of Indian literature. *J Oral Maxillofac Pathol.* 2021;25(2):371-381.
7. Haue MF, Meghji S, Nazir R, Harris M. Interferon gamma may reverse oral submucous fibrosis. *J Oral Pathol Med.* 2001;30(1):12-21.
8. Karbach J, Al-Nawas B, Moergel M, Daubländer M. Oral health-related quality of life of patients with oral lichen planus, oral leukoplakia, or oral squamous cell carcinoma. *J Oral Maxillofac Surg.* 2014;72(8):1517-1522.
9. Diajil AR, Thomson PJ. Risk factors of oral cancer and potentially malignant disorders (PMDs): Developing a high/low risk profiling system. *J Bagh Coll Dent.* 2016;28(3):63-72.
10. Shivhare P, Parihar A. Oral potentially malignant disorder. In: Shivhare P, Parihar A, editors. Textbook of Oral Medicine and Radiology. 2nd ed. Hyderabad: Paras Publisher; 2021. p. 218-58.
11. **Gupta PC, Ray CS.** Smokeless tobacco and health in India and South Asia. *Respirology*. 2003;8(4):419-31.

12. **World Health Organization.** 90% of smokeless tobacco users live in South-East Asia. 2013 Sep 11. Available from: https://www.who.int/southeastasia/news/detail/11-09-2013-90-of-smokeless-tobacco-users-live-in-south-east-asia

13. **Mubeen K, Chandrashekhar H, Kavitha M, Nagarathna S.** Effect of tobacco on oral health: an overview. *J Evol Med Dent Sci.* 2013;2(20):3523-3535.

14. **Xue J, Yang S, Seng S.** Mechanisms of cancer induction by tobacco-specific NNK and NNN. *Cancers (Basel).* 2014;6(2):1138-1156. Available from: https://www.ncbi.nlm.nih.gov/pmc/articles/PMC4074821/

15. Hu, Y., Wang, Y., Chen, Q., Li, Y., Zeng, X., Li, J., & Zhou, Y. (2019). Retinoid treatment for oral leukoplakia: current evidence and future development. *Oral Diseases, 25*(1), 163–171. https://doi.org/10.1111/odi.12802

16. Warnakulasuriya S, Ariyawardana A. "Malignant transformation of oral leukoplakia: a systematic review of observational studies." *Journal of Oral Pathology & Medicine.* 2016;45(3):155-166.

17. Johnson, S.D.; De Costa, A.M.; Young, M.R. Effect of the premalignant and tumor microenvironment on immune cell cytokine production in head and neck cancer. Cancers 2014, 6, 756–770

18. **Bhisey RA.** Chemistry and toxicology of smokeless tobacco. *Indian J Cancer.* 2012;49(4):364-372.

19. **Boffetta P, Hecht S, Gray N, Gupta P, Straif K.** Smokeless tobacco and cancer. *Lancet Oncol.* 2008;9(7):667-675.

20. **Arakeri G, Brennan PA.** Oral submucous fibrosis: an overview of the aetiology, pathogenesis, classification, and principles of management. *Br J Oral Maxillofac Surg.* 2013;51(7):587-593.

21. Johnson, S.D.; De Costa, A.M.; Young, M.R. Effect of the premalignant and tumor microenvironment on immune cell cytokine production in head and neck cancer. Cancers 2014, 6, 756–770

22. **Haue MF, Meghji S, Nazir R, Harris M.** Interferon gamma may reverse oral submucous fibrosis. *J Oral Pathol Med.* 2001;30(1):12-21.

23. **Kumar A, Cascarini L, McCaul JA, Kerawala C, Coombes D, Godden D, Brennan PA.** How should we manage oral leukoplakia? *Br J Oral Maxillofac Surg.* 2013;51(5):377-383.

24. **Arakeri G, Rai KK, Boraks G, et al.** Current protocols in the management of oral submucous fibrosis: an update. *J Oral Pathol Med.* 2017;46(6):418-423. Available from: https://doi.org/10.1111/jop.12583

25. Gauravi A. Mishra, Parishi V. Majmudar, Subhadra D. Gupta, Pallavi S. Rane, PallaviA.Uplap,SurendraS.Shastri.Workplacetobacco cessation program in India:A successstory.Indian J Occup Environ Med. 2009 Dec; 13(3): 146–153

26. World Health Organization, Regional Office for Africa. Types of tobacco use. In: *Tobacco Atlas - 3rd Edition.* 2006. Available from: https://www.afro.who.int/sites/default/files/201709/Chapter%201.%20Types%20of%20tobacco%20use_1.pdf

27. Singh A, Ladusingh L. Prevalence and determinants of tobacco use in India: Evidence from recent Global Adult Tobacco Survey data. PLoS One. 2014;9(12):e114073. journals.plos.org

28. Chauhan N, Paul S, Bhadauria US, Purohit BM, Duggal R, Barma MD, Agarwal D, Bhukal A, Sasidharan S, Shukla P, Khan M, Shenoy R, Malhotra S, Priya H. Investigating the association between tobacco use and oral health among security guards at a tertiary healthcare centre in New Delhi: a cross-sectional study. Front Oral Health. 2024;5:1375792. Frontiers

29. McKinney R, Olmo H. Pathologic manifestations of smokeless tobacco. In: StatPearls. Treasure Island (FL): StatPearls Publishing; 2023.

30. Xu H, Lyu FY, Song JY, Xu YM, Jiang EH, Shang ZJ, et al. Research achievements of oral submucous fibrosis: progress and prospect. Biomed Res Int. 2021;2021:6631856.

31. World Health Organization. Report of a meeting of investigators on the histological definition of precancerous lesions. Geneva: World Health Organization; 1973.

32. Johnson NW. Cancer Biology and Carcinogenesis: Fundamental Biological Processes and How They Are Deranged in Oral Cancer. In: Warnakulasuriya S, Greenspan JS, editors. Textbook of Oral Cancer: Prevention, Diagnosis and Management. Cham: Springer International Publishing; 2020. p. 399-425.

33. Warnakulasuriya S, Kujan O, Aguirre-Urizar JM, Bagan JV, González-Moles MÁ, Kerr AR, Lodi G, Mello FW, Monteiro L, Ogden GR, et al. Oral potentially malignant disorders: A consensus report from an international

seminar on nomenclature and classification, convened by the WHO Collaborating Centre for Oral Cancer. Oral Dis. 2021;27(8):1862-80.

34. Aguirre-Urizar JM. Proliferative multifocal leukoplakia: a better name than proliferative verrucous leukoplakia. World J Surg Oncol. 2011;9:122. doi:10.1186/1477-7819-9-122. PMID: 21943229.

35. Reichart PA, Philipsen HP. Oral erythroplakia—a review. Oral Oncol. 2005;41(6):551-561. doi:10.1016/j.oraloncology.2004.12.003. PMID: 15975518.

36. Kramer IR, Lucas RB, Pindborg JJ, Sobin LH. Definition of leukoplakia and related lesions: an aid to studies on oral precancer. Oral Surg Oral Med Oral Pathol. 1978;46(4):518-39.

37. Kerr AR, Warnakulasuriya S, Mighell AJ, Dietrich T, Nasser M, Gondivkar SM, et al. A systematic review of medical interventions for oral submucous fibrosis and future research opportunities. Oral Dis. 2011;17 Suppl 1:42-57Speight PM, Khurram SA, Kujan O. Oral potentially malignant disorders: risk of progression to malignancy. Oral Surg Oral Med Oral Pathol Oral Radiol. 2018;125(6):612-27.

38. Kramer IR, Lucas RB, Pindborg JJ, Sobin LH. Definition of leukoplakia and related lesions: an aid to studies on oral precancer. Oral Surg Oral Med Oral Pathol. 1978;46(4):518-39.

39. Mortazavi H, Baharvand M, Mehdipour M. Oral potentially malignant disorders: an overview of more than 20 entities. J Dent Res Dent Clin Dent Prospects 2014;8

40. Warnakulasuriya S. Oral potentially malignant disorders: a comprehensive review on clinical aspects and management. *Oral Oncol.* 2020;102:104550. doi:10.1016/j.oraloncology.2020.104550. PMID: 32001133.

41. Reichart PA, Philipsen HP. Oral erythroplakia—a review. Oral Oncol. 2005;41(6):551–561.

42. Pentenero M, Meleti M, Vescovi P, Gandolfo S. Oral proliferative verrucous leukoplakia: Are there particular features for such an ambiguous entity? A systematic review. Br J Dermatol. 2014;170(5):1039-1047. doi: 10.1111/bjd.12797. PMID: 24472098

43. Hansen LS, Olson JA, Silverman S Jr. Proliferative verrucous leukoplakia. A long-term study of thirty patients. Oral Surg Oral Med Oral Pathol. 1985;60(3):285-298. doi:10.1016/0030-4220(85)90313-5. PMID: 3862042

44. Cox SC, Walker DM. Oral submucous fibrosis. A review. Aust Dent J. 1996;41(5):294-9.

45. Warnakulasuriya S. Oral potentially malignant disorders: a comprehensive review on clinical aspects and management. *Oral Oncol.* 2020;102:104550. doi:10.1016/j.oraloncology.2020.104550. PMID: 32001133.

46. Bharath TS, Kumar NG, Nagaraja A, Saraswathi TR, Babu GS, Raju PR. Palatal changes of reverse smokers in a rural coastal Andhra population with review of literature. J Oral Maxillofac Pathol. 2015;19(2):182-7.

47. Jayasooriya, P.R.; Dayaratne, K.; Dissanayake, U.B.; Warnakulasuriya, S. Malignant transformation of oral leukoplakia: a follow-up study. Clin. Oral Investig. 2020, 24(12):4563-4569.

48. Gomez-Armayones S, Chimenos-Kustner E, Mari A, Tous S, Penin R, Clavero O, Quiros B, Pavon MA, Taberna M, Alemany L, et al. Human papillomavirus in premalignant oral lesions: No evidence of association in a Spanish cohort. *PLoS ONE.* 2019;14(1):e0210070. Available from: https://doi.org/10.1371/journal.pone.0210070

49. Ostwald, C., Rutsatz, K., Schweder, J. *et al.* Human papillomavirus 6/11, 16 and 18 in oral carcinomas and benign oral lesions. *Med Microbiol Immunol* **192**, 145–148 (2003).

50. Izumchenko,E.; Sun, K.; Jones, S.; Brait, M.; Agrawal, N.; Koch, W.; McCord, C.L.; Riley, D.R.; Angiuoli, S.V.; Velculescu, V.E.; et al. Notch1 mutations are drivers of oral tumorigenesis. Cancer Prev. Res. 2015, 8, 277–286

51. Johnson, S.D.; De Costa, A.M.; Young, M.R. Effect of the premalignant and tumor microenvironment on immune cell cytokine production in head and neck cancer. Cancers 2014, 6, 756–770

52. Mehanna HM, Rattay T, Smith J, McConkey CC. Treatment and follow up of oral dysplasia - a systematic review and meta-analysis. Head Neck. 2009;31(12):1600-9.

53. Nielsen H, Norrild B, Vedtofte P, Praetorius F, Reibel J, Holmstrup P. Human papillomavirus in oral premalignant lesions. Eur J Cancer B Oral Oncol. 1996;32B(4):264-70.

54. Staines K, Rogers H. Oral leukoplakia and proliferative verrucous leukoplakia: A review for dental practitioners. Br Dent J. 2017;223(9):655-661. doi: 10.1038/sj.bdj.2017.905. PMID: 29151589.
55. Arakeri G, Rai KK, Hunasgi S, Merkx MAW, Gao S, Brennan PA. Oral submucous fibrosis: An update on current theories of pathogenesis. J Oral Pathol Med. 2017;46(6):406-12.
56. Alvarez Gómez GJ, Alvarez Martínez E, Jiménez Gómez R, Mosquera Silva Y, Gaviria Núñez AM, Garcés Agudelo A, et al. Reverse smokers's and changes in oral mucosa. Department of Sucre, Colombia. Med Oral Patol Oral Cir Bucal. 2008;13(1):E1-8
57. Villa, A.; Sonis, S. Oral leukoplakia remains a challenging condition. Oral Dis. 2018, 24, 179–183.
58. Reichart PA, Philipsen HP. Oral erythroplakia--a review. Oral Oncol. 2005;41(6):551-61
59. Rao NR, Villa A, More CB, Jayasinghe RD, Kerr AR, Johnson NW. Oral submucous fibrosis: a contemporary narrative review with a proposed inter-professional approach for an early diagnosis and clinical management. J Otolaryngol Head Neck Surg. 2020;49(1):3
60. Bharath TS, Kumar NG, Nagaraja A, Saraswathi TR, Babu GS, Raju PR. Palatal changes of reverse smokers in a rural coastal Andhra population with review of literature. J Oral Maxillofac Pathol. 2015;19(2):182-7.
61. Ranganathan K, Kavitha L. Oral epithelial dysplasia: Classifications and clinical relevance in risk assessment of oral potentially malignant disorders. J Oral Maxillofac Pathol. 2019;23(1):19-27. doi:10.4103/jomfp.JOMFP_13_19.
62. Bharath TS, Kumar NG, Nagaraja A, Saraswathi TR, Babu GS, Raju PR. Palatal changes of reverse smokers in a rural coastal Andhra population with review of literature. J Oral Maxillofac Pathol. 2015;19(2):182-187. doi:10.4103/0973-029X.164529. PMID: 26604490.
63. Shin D, Vigneswaran N, Gillenwater A, Richards-Kortum R. Advances in fluorescence imaging techniques to detect oral cancer and its precursors. Future Oncol. 2010;6(7):1143-1154. doi:10.2217/fon.10.79
64. Gupta B, Johnson NW. Systematic review and meta-analysis of association of smokeless tobacco and risk of oral cancer in South Asia and the Pacific. PLoS One. 2014;9(11):e113385. doi:10.1371/journal.pone.0113385

65. Shafer WG, Waldron CA. Erythroplakia of the oral cavity. Cancer. 1975;36(3):1021-1028. doi:10.1002/1097-0142(197509)36:3<1021::AID-CNCR2820360327>3.0.CO;2-W
66. Cai X, Yao Z, Liu G, Cui L, Li H, Huang J. Oral submucous fibrosis: A clinicopathological study of 674 cases in China. J Oral Pathol Med. 2019;48(4):321-325. doi:10.1111/jop.12847
67. Abdul NS. Role of advanced diagnostic aids in the detection of potentially malignant disorders and oral cancer at an early stage. Cureus. 2023;15(1):e34113. doi:10.7759/cureus.34113.
68. Lindell G, Eineborg M, Toss G, Karlsson E, Persson B. Silver acetate lozenges in smoking cessation: a double-blind placebo-controlled trial. **Addiction**. 1993;88(4):563–7.
69. Hjalmarson A, Hahn L, Hedner J. Nicotine chewing gum in smoking cessation: a double-blind trial with a placebo. **Clin Pharmacol Ther**. 1979;25(5):563–7.
70. Russell MA, Raw M, Jarvis MJ, Feyerabend C. Nicotine gum as an aid to smoking cessation: a double-blind trial. **Br Med J**. 1980;280(6218):1593–6.
71. Rubinstein ML, Benowitz NL, Auerback GM, Moscicki AB. A randomized trial of nicotine nasal spray in adolescent smokers; Pediatrics.2008 Sep; 122(3):e595-600
72. Jarvis MJ, Raw M, Russell MA, Feyerabend C. Randomised controlled trial of nicotine chewing-gum as an adjunct to group therapy in smoking cessation. **Br Med J (Clin Res Ed)**. 1982;285(6341):537–40.
73. Daughton DM, Heatley SA, Prendergast JJ, Williams HL, Puska P, Kunos G. Effectiveness of nicotine chewing gum as an adjunct to physician's advice and support in smoking cessation. **JAMA**. 1986;256(10):1310–3.
74. Arcori L, Proctor CJ, Tucker A, Wadsworth D, Green M. The acute thermogenic effects of chewing gum containing different doses of nicotine and caffeine. **Eur J Clin Nutr**. 1994;48(7):545-53
75. Leigh R, Viner NM, CoxG, Balon JW, Wilson DM, O'Shaughnessy D, et al. Nicotine replacement combined with a novel compound (ProBAN) for smoking cessation: a pilot study. Can Respir J 2001; 8(1):21-6.
76. Oncken C, Dornelas E. Nicotine gum for pregnant smokers: a randomized controlled trial.; Obstet Gynecol. 2008 Oct;112(4):859-67

77. Christen A, Beiswanger B, Mau M, Walker C, Hatsukami D, Allen S, et al. Transdermal Nicotine for Smoking Cessation JAMA. 1991; 266(22):3133-3138.
78. Otero UB, Perez Cde A, Szklo M, Esteves GA, dePinho MM, Szklo AS, et al. Randomized clinical trial: effectiveness of the cognitive-behavioral approach and the use of nicotine replacement transdermal patches for smoking cessation among adults in Riode Janeiro, Brazil; Cad Saude Publica. 2006 Feb; 22(2):439-49.
79. Yudkin P L, Jones L, Lancaster T, Fowler G H. Which smokers are helped to give up smoking using transdermal nicotine patches? Results from a randomized, double-blind, placebo controlled trial. British Journal of General Practice 1996; 46:145-148.
80. Ebbert JO, Post JA, Moyer TP, Dale LC, Schroeder DR, Hurt RD. Nicotine percentage replacement among smokeless tobacco users with nicotine patch; Drug Alcohol Depend. 2007 Jul 10;89(2-3):223-6.
81. David SP, Munafò MR, Murphy MF, Proctor M, Walton RT, Johnstone EC. Genetic variation in the dopamine D4 receptor (DRD4) gene and smoking cessation: follow-up of a randomised clinical trial of transdermal nicotine patch; Pharmacogenomics J. 2008 Apr; 8(2):122-8.
82. Shafer WG, Waldron CA. Erythroplakia of the oral cavity. Cancer. 1975;36(3):1021-1028. doi:10.1002/1097-0142(197509)36:3<1021::AID-CNCR2820360327>3.0.CO;2-W
83. Arakeri G, Rai KK, Boraks G, Patil SG, Aljabab AS, Merkx MAW, et al. Current protocols in the management of oral submucous fibrosis: An update. J Oral Pathol Med. 2017;46(6):418-23.
84. Russell MA, Stapleton JA, Feyerabend C, Wiseman SM, Gustavsson G, Sawe U, et al. Targeting heavy smokers in general practice: randomised controlled trial of transdermal nicotine patches; BMJ 1993;306;1308-12.
85. Glenn IM, Dallery J. Effects of internet-based voucher reinforcement and a transdermal nicotine patch on cigarette smoking; J Appl Behav Anal. 2007 Spring; 40(1):1-13.
86. Benowitz NL, Zevin S, Jacob P 3rd. Suppression of Nicotine Intake During Ad Libitum Cigarette Smoking by High-Dose Transdermal Nicotine. JPET 1998; 287:958–962.

87. Hatsukami D, Mooney M, Murphy S, LeSage M, Babb D, Hecht S. Effects of high dose transdermal nicotine replacementin cigarette smokers; Pharmacol Biochem Behav. 2007 Jan; 86(1):132-9.

88. Dale LC, Schroeder DR, Wolter TD, Croghan IT, Hurt RD, Offord KP.Weight change after smoking cessation using variable doses of transdermal nicotine replacement. J Gen Intern Med 1998; 13(1): 9-15.

89. Shaw JP, Ferry DG, Pethica D, Brenner D, Tucker IG. Usage patterns of transdermal nicotine when purchased as a non-prescription medicine from Pharmacies. Tobacco Control 1998; 7:161–167.

90. Abu-Huwaij R, Obaidat RM, Sweidan K, Al-Hiari Y. Formulation and in vitro evaluation of xanthan gum or carbopol 934 based mucoadhesive patches, loaded with nicotine; AAPS PharmSciTech.2011 Mar;12(1):21-7.

91. Tang JL, Law M, Wald N. How effective is nicotine replacement therapy inhelping people to stop smoking? BMJ 1994; 308:21-6.

92. Cooney NL, Cooney JL. Smoking cessation during alcohol treatment: a randomized trial of combination nicotine patch plus nicotine gum; Addiction. 2009 Sep; 104(9):1588-96.

93. Russell MA, Jarvis MJ, Feyerabend C, Fernö O. Nasal nicotine solution:a potential aid to giving up smoking? BMJ 1983; 286: 683-684.

94. Tonnesen P, Nørregaard J, Mikkelsen K, Jorgensen S, Nilsson F. A Double-blind Trial of a Nicotine Inhaler for Smoking Cessation. JAMA 1993; 269:1268- 1271.

95. Kralikova E, Kozak JT, Smoking cessation or reduction with nicotine replacement therapy: a placebo-controlled double blind trial with nicotine gum and inhaler; BMCPublic Health. 2009 Nov 27; 9:433

96. Hand S, Edwards S, Campbell IA, Cannings R. Controlled trial of three weeks nicotine replacement treatment in hospital patients also given advice and support; Thorax. 2002 Aug;57(8):715-8

97. Fagerström K O , Hughes J R , Rasmussen T, Callas P W. Randomised trial investigating effect of a novel nicotine delivery device(Eclipse) and a nicotine oral inhaler on smoking behaviour, nicotine and carbon monoxide exposure, and motivation to quit. Tobacco Control 2000; 9:327–333.

98. Rey L, Vaucher P, Secretan F, Zellweger JP, Bodenmann P. Use of nicotine substitute prescribed at hourly plus ad libitum intake or ad libitum for heavy

smokers willing to quit: a randomized controlled trial; Subst Abuse Treat PrevPolicy. 2009 Jun 2;4:12

99. Hajek P, West R, Foulds J Nilsson F, Burrows S, Meadow A. Randomized Comparative Trial of Nicotine Polacrilex, a Transdermal Patch, Nasal Spray, and an Inhaler. Arch Intern Med 1999; 159:2033-2038.

100. Rubinstein ML, Benowitz NL, Auerback GM, Moscicki AB. A randomized trial of nicotine nasal spray in adolescent smokers; Pediatrics.2008 Sep; 122(3):e595-600

101. Rabius V, Pike KJ, Hunter J, Wiatrek D, McAlister AL. Effects of frequency and duration in telephone counselling for smoking cessation. Tob Control. 2007Dec;16 Suppl 1(Suppl 1):i71-4.

102. Warnakulasuriya S, Kujan O, Aguirre-Urizar JM, Bagan JV, González-Moles MÁ, Kerr AR, et al. Oral potentially malignant disorders: A consensus report from an international seminar on nomenclature and classification. *Oral Dis.* 2021;27(8):1862-1880.

103. Rai V, Mukherjee R, Gadre A, Chatterjee K, Bhowmik K, Datta S. Role of antioxidants in oral potentially malignant disorders and oral squamous cell carcinoma: A review. *J Oral Biol Craniofac Res.* 2021;11(2):175-181. Available from: https://www.ncbi.nlm.nih.gov/pmc/articles/PMC5603668/

104. Trejo-Solís C, Pedraza-Chaverrí J, Torres-Ramos M, Jiménez-Farfán D, Cruz-Salgado A, Serrano-García N, et al. Multiple molecular and cellular mechanisms of action of lycopene in cancer inhibition. *Evid Based Complement Alternat Med.* 2013;2013:705121. Available from: https://www.ncbi.nlm.nih.gov/pmc/articles/PMC3714846

105. Karemore, T., Motwani, M., Motghare, P., Dalal, S., Panchbhai, A., & Banubakode, T. (2020). Efficacy of lycopene in the management of oral leukoplakia – A systematic review. *Journal of Oral and Maxillofacial Pathology, 24*(1), 143–150. https://doi.org/10.4103/jomfp.JOMFP_101_19

106. **Singh M, Krishanappa R, Bagewadi A, Keluskar V.** Efficacy of oral lycopene in the treatment of oral leukoplakia. *Oral Oncol.* 2004;40(6):591-596.

107. Gopinath, D., Hui, L. M., Veettil, S. K., Nair, A. B., & Maharajan, M. K. (2022). Comparative efficacy of interventions for the management of oral submucous fibrosis: A systematic review and network meta-analysis. *Journal of Personalized Medicine, 12*(8), 1272. https://doi.org/10.3390/jpm12081272

108. Saini, R., Ahuja, U. S., Puri, N., Rathore, A., Ahuja, S., & Das, S. R. (2022). Comparative evaluation of lycopene and therapeutic ultrasound by using diagnostic ultrasonography in the management of oral submucous fibrosis (OSMF): A clinical trial. *Journal of Clinical and Diagnostic Research, 16*(3), ZC01-ZC05. doi:10.7860/JCDR/2022/49398.

109. Nagao, T., Warnakulasuriya, S., Nakamura, T., Kato, S., Yamamoto, K., Fukano, H., Suzuki, K., Shimozato, K., & Hashimoto, S. (2015). Treatment of oral leukoplakia with a low-dose of beta-carotene and vitamin C supplements: A randomized controlled trial. *International Journal of Cancer, 136*(7), 1708–1717. https://doi.org/10.1002/ijc.29160

110. Lodi G, Franchini R, Warnakulasuriya S, Varoni EM, Sardella A, Kerr AR, Carrassi A, MacDonald LCI, Worthington HV. Interventions for treating oral leukoplakia to prevent oral cancer. Cochrane Database of Systematic Reviews 2016, Issue 7. Art. No.: CD001829

111. Nilesh, K., Dadhich, A., Saluja, H., Patil, D., & Vande, A. (2020). Treatment of oral submucous fibrosis with lycopene, beta-carotene, zinc, selenium, copper, alpha-lipoic acid, and alpha-tocopheryl acetate: A randomized controlled trial. *Journal of Oral and Maxillofacial Surgery, 78*(5), 767.e1-767.e7.

112. See, J. K. L., Liu, X., Canfora, F., Moore, C., McCullough, M., Yap, T., Paolini, R., & Celentano, A. (2021). The role of vitamins in oral potentially malignant disorders and oral cancer: A systematic review. *Oral Diseases, 27*(1), 197–210. https://doi.org/10.1111/odi.13356

113. Islam, M., Ali, M. N., Anwar, R. B., Asaduzzaman, M., Islam, A. S. M. A., Hussain, M., & Rahman, Q. B. (2023). The role of Vitamin A, Vitamin C, and Vitamin E for chemoprevention of oral leukoplakia. *International Journal of Contemporary Medical Research, 10*(1), 1–8.

114. Sune, R. V., Bhowate, R. R., Lohe, V. K., & Dangore-Khasbage, S. B. (2024). Role of antioxidant vitamins in oral submucous fibrosis: A narrative review. *Cureus, 16*(5), e59596.

115. Nallapu, V., Balasankulu, B., Vuppalapati, H. B., Sambhana, S., Mala, D., & Koppula, S. K. (2015). Efficacy of vitamin E in oral submucous fibrosis: A clinical and histopathologic study. *Journal of Indian Academy of Oral Medicine and Radiology, 27*(3), 387-392.

116. Hu, Y., Wang, Y., Chen, Q., Li, Y., Zeng, X., Li, J., & Zhou, Y. (2019). Retinoid treatment for oral leukoplakia: current evidence and future development. *Oral Diseases, 25*(1), 163–171. https://doi.org/10.1111/odi.12802

117. Poveda-Roda, R., Bagán, J. V., Jiménez-Soriano, Y., Díaz-Fernández, J. M., & Gavaldá-Esteve, C. (2010). Retinoids and proliferative verrucous leukoplakia (PVL): A preliminary study. *Medicina Oral, Patología Oral y Cirugía Bucal, 15*(6), e872–e875.

118. Kulkarni, R., Kalaskar, A., Kalaskar, R., & Gupta, N. (2020). Efficacy of spirulina in management of oral submucous fibrosis: A systematic review. *Journal of Oral Medicine and Radiology, 7*(2), 53–58. https://doi.org/10.4103/jomr.jomr_25_20

119. Kumar, K. R., Sravanthi, Y. M., Suresh, D., Avinash, K., Khandare, S., & Pavana, M. H. (2022). Comparative evaluation of the chemoprevention of oral leukoplakia with spirulina and green tea extract. *International Journal of Contemporary Medical Research, 9*(11), K1–K5.

120. Kuriakose, M. A., Ramdas, K., Dey, B., Iyer, S., Rajan, G., Elango, K. K., Suresh, A., Ravindran, D., Kumar, R. R., Prathiba, R., Ramachandran, S., Kumar, N. A., Thomas, G., Somanathan, T., Ravindran, H. K., Ranganathan, K., Katakam, S. B., Parashuram, S., Jayaprakash, V., & Pillai, M. R. (2016). A randomized double-blind placebo-controlled Phase IIB trial of curcumin in oral leukoplakia. *Cancer Prevention Research, 9*(8), 683–691. https://doi.org/10.1158/1940-6207.CAPR-15-0409

121. Vijayalaxmi N, Reddy RS, Ramesh T, Saimadhavi N, Reddy RL, Swapna LA. Efficacy of curcumin in treating palatal changes associated with reverse smoking. J Oral Maxillofac Pathol. 2015;19(3):344-350. doi:10.4103/0973-029X.174624. PMID: 26980964.

122. She, R., & Xu, P. (2024). Mechanism of curcumin in the prevention and treatment of oral submucosal fibrosis and progress in clinical application research. *Journal of Clinical Medicine, 13*(4), 1103. https://doi.org/10.3390/jcm13041103

123. Gopinath, D., Hui, L. M., Veettil, S. K., Nair, A. B., & Maharajan, M. K. (2022). Comparative efficacy of interventions for the management of oral submucous fibrosis: A systematic review and network meta-analysis. *Journal of Personalized Medicine, 12*(8), 1272. https://doi.org/10.3390/jpm12081272

124. Kataria S, Sahoo S, Marya CM, Nagpal R, Taneja P. Aged garlic extract as a wonder herb in medicine and oral care: A comprehensive review. J Indian Assoc Public Health Dent. 2023;21(4):288-293.

125. Armstrong, W. B., Taylor, T. H., Kennedy, A. R., Melrose, R. J., Messadi, D. V., Gu, M., Le, A. D., Perloff, M., Civantos, F., Goodwin, W. J., Wirth, L. J., Kerr, A. R., & Meyskens, F. L. Jr. (2013). Bowman Birk Inhibitor Concentrate and Oral Leukoplakia: A Randomized Phase IIb Trial. *Cancer Prevention Research, 6*(5), 410–418. https://doi.org/10.1158/1940-6207.CAPR-13-0004

126. Lodi G, Sardella A, Bez C, Demarosi F, Carrassi A. Systematic review of randomized trials for the treatment of oral leukoplakia. *J Dent Educ.* 2002;66(8):896-902.

127. Saba, N. F., Hurwitz, S. J., Kono, S. A., Yang, C. S., Zhao, Y., Chen, Z., Lewis, M., Morris, J., Shin, D. M., & Khuri, F. R. (2014). Chemoprevention of Head and Neck Cancer with Celecoxib and Erlotinib: Results of a Phase Ib and Pharmacokinetic Study. *Cancer Prevention Research, 7*(3), 283–291. https://doi.org/10.1158/1940-6207.CAPR-13-0243

128. Liu, J., Chen, F., Wei, Z., Qiu, M., Li, Z., Dan, H., Chen, Q., & Jiang, L. (2017). Evaluating the efficacy of pentoxifylline in the treatment of oral submucous fibrosis: A meta-analysis. *Oral Diseases, 23*(8), 1023–1032. https://doi.org/10. 1111/ odi.12715

129. Chen, X., Xie, H. & Guo, J. Drug treatment for oral submucous fibrosis: an update. *BMC Oral Health* **23**, 748 (2023). https://doi.org/10.1186/s12903-023-03488-9

130. Chen, X., Xie, H., & Guo, J. (2023). Drug treatment for oral submucous fibrosis: An update. *BMC Oral Health, 23*(1), 748. https://doi.org/10.1186/s 12903-023-03488-9

131. Staines, K., & Rogers, H. (2017). Proliferative verrucous leukoplakia: A general dental practitioner-focused clinical review. *Primary Dental Journal, 6*(2), 40–43.

132. Townsend M, Kejner AE, Nourollah-Zadeh F, et al. Eradication of proliferative verrucous leukoplakia with toll-like receptor 7 agonist (topical imiquimod): a case report. Front Oncol. 2024;14:1473889. doi:10.3389/fonc.2024.1473889.

133. Shinge AA, Kanchan T, Talreja D, Kumar N, Bhagchandani J, Shetty S. Comparative evaluation of the efficacy of systemic levamisole and antioxidant in the management of oral submucous fibrosis – A randomized control trial. J Adv Clin Res Insights. 2019;6(3):91-95.

134. Shen, Y. W., Shih, Y. H., Fuh, L. J., & Shieh, T. M. (2020). Oral submucous fibrosis: A review on biomarkers, pathogenic mechanisms, and treatments. *Cancers, 12*(10), 3022. https://doi.org/10.3390/cancers12103022

135. Rao NR, Arakeri G, Brennan PA, Kailasam S, Jafer M, Warnakulasuriya S. The role of intralesional interferon-gamma in the management of oral submucous fibrosis: A systematic review. *J Oral Pathol Med.* 2017;46(6):413-421. doi:10.1111/jop.12580.

136. Shetty, S. R., Al-Bayati, S. A. A. F., & Shon, A. A. (2013). Bleomycin chemotherapy for oral leukoplakia. *Journal of Cancer Research and Therapeutics, 9*(4), 571–574. https://doi.org/10.4103/0973-1482.126474

137. Tsao, A. S., Liu, D., Martin, J., Tang, X. M., Lee, J. J., El-Naggar, A. K., Wistuba, I. I., Culotta, K. S., Mao, L., Gillenwater, A., & Lippman, S. M. (2021). Inhibition of mTOR signaling and clinical activity of metformin in oral premalignant lesions. *JCI Insight, 6*(1), e147096. https://doi.org/10.1172/jci.insight.147096

138. Shah, P. H., Venkatesh, R., More, C. B., & Vassandacoumara, V. (2016). Comparison of therapeutic efficacy of placental extract with dexamethasone and hyaluronic acid with dexamethasone for oral submucous fibrosis: A retrospective analysis. *Journal of Clinical and Diagnostic Research, 10*(10), ZC63-ZC66. doi:10.7860/JCDR/2016/8652.8652.

139. Patil, S., Maheshwari, S., & Khandelwal, S. (2018). Comparative evaluation of placental extract and intralesional steroids in oral submucous fibrosis. *Indian Journal of Dental Research, 29*(3), 321-327

140. Lin HJ, Lin JC. Treatment of oral submucous fibrosis by collagenase: effects on oral opening and eating function. Oral Dis. 2007;13(4):407-413. doi:10.1111/j.1601-0825.2006.01313.x. PMID: 17577328.

141. Chitlange, N. M., & Phansopkar, P. (2023). Physiotherapeutic approach in oral submucous fibrosis: A systematic review. *Cureus, 15*(11), e48155. https://doi.org/10.7759/cureus.48155

142. Senthilkumar, S., Chitra, S., Vijayaraghavan, R., Hemaashree, V., & Subhavani, P. (2021). Effectiveness of ultrasound therapy on oral submucosal fibrosis. *Journal of Physical Therapy Science, 33*(10), 850–855. https://doi.org/10.1589/jpts.33.850

143. Chandran, V., Reddy, R. S., Ramesh, T., & Kumar, B. N. (2017). Use of mouth opening screws in the management of oral submucous fibrosis: A clinical evaluation. *Journal of Oral and Maxillofacial Surgery, 75*(1), 35-40.

144. Sharma, S., Gupta, D. S., & Thomas, R. (2020). Mouth opening screws in the treatment of oral submucous fibrosis: A randomized controlled trial. *Oral Surgery, Oral Medicine, Oral Pathology, and Oral Radiology, 130*(6), 681-687.

145. Mehta, D., Desai, V., & Patel, K. (2021). Combination of mouth opening screws and corticosteroid therapy in oral submucous fibrosis. *Journal of Oral Science, 63*(1), 53-59.

146. Singh, A., Kumar, V., & Gupta, R. (2023). Challenges in using mouth opening screws in advanced oral submucous fibrosis. *International Journal of Oral and Maxillofacial Surgery, 52*(3), 367-373.

147. Bhattarai BP, Singh AK, Singh RP, Chaulagain R, Søland TM, Hasséus B, Sapkota D. Recurrence in Oral Leukoplakia: A Systematic Review and Meta-analysis. J Dent Res. 2024 Oct;103(11):1066-1075. doi: 10.1177/00220345241266519. Epub 2024 Sep 18. PMID: 39290142; PMCID: PMC11504345.

148. Luo R, Wang Y, Li R, et al. Laser therapy decreases oral leukoplakia recurrence and boosts patient comfort: a network meta-analysis and systematic review. BMC Oral Health. 2024;24(1):469. doi:10.1186/s12903-024-04179-9.

149. Cobb CM, Beaini NE, Scully J, Gibson TM. Proliferative verrucous leukoplakia: Case study of 24 years and outcome of treatment with CO_2 laser. Clin Adv Periodontics. 2024 Oct;14(4):e1-e8. doi: 10.1002/cap.10320.

150. Bombeccari GP, Garagiola U, Candotto V, Pallotti F, Carinci F, Giannì AB, Spadari F. Diode laser surgery in the treatment of oral proliferative verrucous leukoplakia associated with HPV-16 infection. Maxillofac Plast Reconstr Surg. 2018;40(1):16. doi: 10.1186/s40902-018-0156-2. PMID: 29770153; PMCID: PMC5951821.

151. Condor D, Culcițchi C, Blum R, Baru O, Buduru S, Kui A, Țig I. A Review of CO_2 Laser-Mediated Therapy for Oral Mucosal Lesions. Appl Sci. 2021;11(16):7744. doi: 10.3390/app11167744.

152. Sattayut S, Srisilapanan P, Patcharanuchat P. Utilizing laser therapy to manage oral potentially malignant disorders in older adults at the primary care level. Adv Clin Exp Med. 2024;33(10):1033-1042. doi: 10.17219/acem/176588.

153. Gondivkar SM, Gadbail AR, Sarode SC, Gondivkar RS, Patil S, Gaikwad RN, Chu DT, Yuwanati M. Treatment outcomes of laser therapy in oral submucous fibrosis: a systematic review. J Oral Biol Craniofac Res. 2020 Jul-Sep;10(3):253-258. doi: 10.1016/j.jobcr.2020.05.004. PMID: 32518740; PMCID: PMC7278429.

154. Aparna TY, Pushpanjali M, Aruna P, Fathima PR, Vishal AJ, Mala D. Evaluation of the efficacy of laser biostimulation and intralesional corticosteroids in the management of oral submucous fibrosis: A comparative study. J Indian Acad Oral Med Radiol. 2023;35(2):120-125. doi: 10.4103/jiaomr.jiaomr_70_23.

155. Kumar, Varun; Malhotra, Divye[1]; Mular, Ashish G.[2]; Sachan, Swapnil[3]; Sharma, Deepali[3]. Cryosurgery for the Treatment of Oral Leukoplakia: Satisfying or Not?. Indian Journal of Dental Sciences 9(4):p 256-260, Oct–Dec 2017. | DOI: 10.4103/IJDS.IJDS_73_17

156. Pandey A, Kaur S, Ashem A, Sarin S, Sahu RK, Jadav BP, Mehta DN, Makkad RS. Cryotherapy for oral potentially malignant disorders. Bioinformation. 2023;19(13):1377-1382. doi: 10.6026/973206300191377

157. Liu W, Yang X, Shi L, Shen X. Surgery management of oral cavity premalignancy needs risk stratification and randomized controlled trials

158. Abadie, W.M.; Partington, E.J.; Fowler, C.B.; Schmalbach, C.E. Optimal Management of Proliferative Verrucous Leukoplakia: A Systematic Review of the Literature. Otolaryngol. - Head Neck Surg. (United States) 2015, 153, 504–511

159. Awadallah, M.; Idle, M.; Patel, K.; Kademani, D. Management update of potentially premalignant oral epithelial lesions. Oral Surg. Oral Med. Oral Pathol. Oral Radiol. 2018, 125, 628–636

FSC
www.fsc.org
MIX
Papier | Fördert
gute Waldnutzung
FSC® C083411

Kolibri 360 GmbH
Ferdinand-Jühlke-Straße 7
99095 Erfurt, Deutschland
produktsicherheit@kolibri360.de

Druck:
CPI Druckdienstleistungen GmbH
im Auftrag der
Kolibri 360 GmbH
Ferdinand-Jühlke-Str. 7
99095 Erfurt